Reproducing Inequities

Reproducing Inequities

Poverty and the Politics of Population in Haiti

M. CATHERINE MATERNOWSKA

With a Foreword by Paul Farmer

RUTGERS UNIVERSITY PRESS

NEW BRUNSWICK, NEW JERSEY, AND LONDON

LIBRARY OF CONGRESS CATALOGING-IN-PUBLICATION DATA

Maternowska, M. Catherine, 1961–
    Reproducing inequities : poverty and the politics of population in Haiti /
M. Catherine Maternowska.
        p.   cm.—(Rutgers studies in medical anthropology)
    Includes bibliographical references and index.
    ISBN-13-978-0-8135-3853-2 (hardcover : alk. paper) — ISBN-13-978-0-8135-3854-9
(pbk : alk. paper)
    1. Poverty—Haiti.   2. Haiti—Population policy.   3. Haiti—Economic
conditions—1971.   I. Title.   II. Series: Rutgers series in medical anthropology.
    HC153.Z9P65   2006
    362.5097294—dc22   2005028037
                                                                          CIP

A British Cataloging-in-Publication record for this book is available
from the British Library.

Manufactured in the United States of America

To my sources of love and inspiration,
on both sides of the Atlantic Ocean–
Caleb, Malcolm, and Alexander Duncan,
and the people of Cité Soleil.

CONTENTS

FOREWORD

Unraveling Fertility and Power

PAUL FARMER

Poverty and social inequalities, including gender inequality, have become increasingly important as subjects of study for anthropologists. But no book better explores the painful intersection of these subjects with ethnographic depth and theoretical rigor than Catherine Maternowska's new study of family planning in one of the poorest slums in the world—Haiti's Cité Soleil. *Reproducing Inequities: Poverty and the Politics of Population in Haiti* is much more than a study of the vicissitudes of Haitian women seeking to control fertility in a setting where they cannot easily feed or protect their children. It is a painful and harrowing exploration of how aid programs purporting to reduce fertility come to fail their poorest "clients," to use a telling bit of family planning jargon. And fail they have, even though family planning efforts have been supported generously by the U.S. Agency for International Development (USAID) and the International Planned Parenthood Federation (IPPF), two of the largest funders in the field:

> By Western Hemisphere standards, Haiti's progress in family planning is at best very poor. Even if contraceptive prevalence climbed approximately 4 percent during the period under study, it did not affect overall fertility rates, and there has been a general failure to achieve better health and quality of life for women, men, and children. Three decades since the population control sector's inception, the institutions that usurped control of the public sector—including USAID, IPPF, the Population Council, and several others—were still actively working in Haiti in the 1990s. A great proportion of their work was spent determining why family planning efforts have failed so markedly but, ultimately, their efforts to effect change have been minimal.

These failures lead to great death and disability, almost all of it registered among women living in poverty. Haiti's example is dire. One 2001 report cited in *Reproducing Inequities* surveys over 130 countries and reveals that, after more than two decades of effort and tens of millions of dollars of investment, Haiti remains the only Western-hemisphere country in the "high-risk" category, as far as pregnancy and childbirth go. Another study cited by Maternowska pegs maternal mortality in Haiti at about the highest in the world. But middle-class Haitian women suffer rates of maternal death that differ little from those of their economic peers elsewhere in the world. Central to this problem are, of course, poor women's lack of access to modern obstetrics, but also low rates of contraceptive use.

So why don't more Haitians use modern contraception? It takes an experienced and exceptionally committed anthropologist, perhaps, to answer this question honestly and compellingly.

Since Maternowska's book offers a comprehensive overview of recent demographic studies of Haiti, what some have termed Haiti's "fertility paradox" emerges clearly from her survey. *Reproducing Inequities* teaches us that, in spite of a widespread desire among Haitian women to have fewer children, and in spite of at least official support from various Haitian governments and their funders to the north, fertility rates have remained high and unchanged. Unraveling this paradox is a primary goal of this study, and Maternowska dismisses, one by one, the standard, easy explanations. Was it because there were no funds committed to family planning? Maternowska shows us that the answer to this question is no, even though investments in improving access to other services, including modern obstetrics, were often scant. By the late twentieth century, Haiti received twice as much family planning assistance as any other country in the hemisphere: "Funding continued to flood the sector; by 1988 the family planning sector alone was valued at thirteen and a half million dollars." This study shows how USAID's support for family planning ballooned over the course of a decade in which Haiti's fertility rate actually increased.

Similarly dismissed are culturalist explanations, which receive heavy play whenever powerful planners and funders are faced with the obstinate fact that well-laid plans often go astray among the poorest. As has been seen with other persistent health problems, in the realm of fertility medicine, those not themselves living in poverty are quick to ascribe program failure to clients' "ignorance" or "cultural beliefs." Such explanations, though seldom buttressed by data, are rife in development work in general. *Underdevelopment Is a State of Mind*, by Lawrence Harrison (who was himself the ranking USAID official in Haiti during at least part of the period described by Maternowska), stands as one classic example of this sort of analysis, which gives short shrift to history and political economy and admits almost no consideration of the adverse impact of colonial and neocolonial policies, to say nothing of racism or gender inequality. The result of such desocialization, in development circles and in international health programs, is typically recourse to victim blaming. But Maternowska's study suggests that lack of knowledge—ignorance—about family planning is far from the top of the list of explanations of the Haitian paradox: "The women and men of Cité Soleil know far better than any development experts the terrible costs of having and raising children in such wretched conditions."

If victim blaming is to be eschewed and sound analysis of such failures is an urgent priority, what framework might enable us to understand why, if Haitian women know about and want to use contraception, investments in contraception have failed to produce the desired results? To answer this question, Maternowska uses several frameworks and many approaches. She grounds her ethnographic analysis in what is termed, again in the jargon of demography, the "political economy of fertility." But to these "macro" understandings of demography and political economy, an intrepid and persistent anthropologist can add much more. Maternowska's interviews, whether structured or open-ended, and her observations of life in the dangerous tumult of Cité Soleil, show us again and again how difficult it is to provide decent family planning services, much less comprehensive women's health care, in the midst of enormous political upheaval. During one of the darkest periods in which this research was conducted, the clinic she studied was closed two weeks out of the month. This did not stop some of those running this and other clinics from blaming their "clients" for their own inability to "comply" with the contraceptive regimes advocated by those in charge.

Perhaps only an anthropologist like Catherine Maternowska could obtain this sort of information, intimate knowledge solicited from the powerful and the disenfranchised. Certainly this is a book that could only be written by a mature anthropologist—perhaps only one with two decades of research experience in Haiti and, perhaps more to the point, with two decades of concern for the poorest citizens of that country. Each chapter is leavened with intimate detail that is at once respectful and revealing. Maternowska is a true participant-observer, honest about her own different modes of involvement—she worked largely for the family planning programs she critiques—and about the ways in which her involvement was understood by Haitians, rich and poor alike, men and women alike.

Reproducing Inequities is beautifully written, with ethnographic vignettes that give us the texture and feel—and even the unwelcome smells and noises— of a rapidly expanding, informal settlement, the largest and poorest in Haiti. Cité Soleil is a tightly packed slum with neighborhoods like "Cardboard City." It is peopled largely by landless peasants and their children. They work, if they are lucky enough to work, as domestic servants, street vendors, or day laborers; some even have jobs in the offshore assembly industry that permits U.S. and Asian firms to bypass the organized labor of more affluent countries. Most are unemployed and must rely for survival on their connections to someone—kin or a partner—with a job. Maternowska is unflinchingly straightforward about the impact of this on sexual histories: "Women's power in the realm of sexuality is almost always directed toward financial gain. Every woman interviewed told me they were not in a relationship for love of sexual enjoyment. Rather, unions help women survive." Poor Haitians have long struggled back, and valiantly, against precisely these sorts of conditions and the "structures of feeling" they generate.

Most of Maternowska's fieldwork was conducted during periods of great political change and upheaval. An understanding of the trials of the Haitian popular movement, with strong bases in Cité Soleil and other slums, constitutes one of the major plotlines of the story. This struggle, like almost all others in the poorer reaches of the world, is gendered. Even the metaphors are gendered, as Maternowska reminds us in discussing, dryly enough, "the abortive presidential elections" of 1987 and the military and paramilitary disorder that followed. But the author never strays from her topic of how and why family planning efforts fail. To push such metaphors further, a political economy of fertility, one alive to social process, is where the rubber meets the road for those who seek to understand why programs such as those studied here fail to protect the lives and the rights of women living in poverty. Maternowska does not simply note the complex interplay of fertility and power; she describes in heartbreaking detail how "local" gendered relations and translocal social processes have helped to shape everything from the definition of Haiti's policies to whether or not there would be stock-outs of such deliverables as condoms or oral contraceptives. *Reproducing Inequities* reveals how gender inequality, deep poverty, and political violence are *embodied* in the poor health outcomes of the poorest.

Maternowska's book draws on many disciplines, but it is above all an anthropological study. With informants from all strata of Haitian society and from within the powerful institutions dictating policy, she "studies up" and "studies down," cutting what Laura Nader would call a "vertical slice" through one of the most ideology-laden of topics. It is part insider's account of the foreign-aid machine, part memoir, and part ethnography. Maternowska notes: "As a longtime resident in the community, as well as frequent visitor to and observer of the offices of USAID, I was privy to the heated political debates about health care delivery from the perspective of the poor as well as that of the powerful." In a sharp characterization of funders and policy makers—largely from USAID, but from other agencies as well—Maternowska reports that "consultants called on to assist are typically isolated from Haiti's reality from the moment they deplane." In addition to the politicization of aid and health care decisions by the powerful in Washington and Port-au-Prince, with ripples felt sharply among the poor, there is also the consultants' simple lack of proximity to those ostensibly served. For example, one high-ranking official within the aid bureaucracy, charged with family planning, "lived in Haiti for nearly five years before he ever entered the site that housed a former Cité Soleil family planning clinic funded by the agency—and that was after persistent urging on my part." In order to accomplish what she terms "laptop report analysis and writing by U.S. consultants," consultants move between comfortable retreats in the cool hills far above Cité Soleil and the offices of USAID: "A huge fortresslike wall keeps government employees safely sealed in, and out of sight. Those entering must undergo perfunctory car searches as a preliminary security check. The offices are housed in what was once the Beau Rivage, a lovely tropical hotel . . . visitors cross a tiny footbridge (with koi swimming below) to enter into the icy cold, air-conditioned interior of the agency." By "government employees," Maternowska means U.S. government employees, and one of the achievements of her study is to reveal how development bureaucracies can lose their grasp on the problems they came to solve, in spite of the best intentions of many of those cloistered within this and other cool fortresses across the world. What she writes about USAID holds too for similar agencies—French and British equivalents, the European Union writ large, and also the World Bank and the International Monetary Fund—that together control the fates, and not merely the reproductive trajectories, of millions of the world's poorest citizens.

Maternowska is brave enough to share information that will win her few friends within these underperforming institutions. Some of her informants among Haitian professionals are likely to take umbrage as well. But it is important that those seeking to improve services to the poor understand how class works in a society traversed by such steep grades of inequality. The victim blaming apparent among some of the development set is not an expatriate specialty. Middle-class Haitian nurses, for example, were quick to pin the blame for program failure on the culture of poverty. One Haitian physician actually made a reference, during a clinical session and in front of a patient, to C.L.R. James's classic study of the Haitian revolution, explaining later that the patient's unwelcome behavior was just like that of the slaves: "Those slaves they were stupid and they lied. They could easily hold you in their lies." As Maternowska tersely notes, the doctor misquoted James, and certainly missed the spirit of his account, which relayed the fecklessness and cruelty of the slavemasters. "Like the master in the literary passage, the doctor, during his consultation, failed to admit his own mistake and punished the client for it, denying her her preferred method of contraception or a reasonable alternative."

Maternowska supplies, alas, many such anecdotes. In her book, however, it is the voices of the poor that dominate. The interviews push us into the realm of symbolic anthropology, because Maternowska explores the meanings of family planning efforts among their intended beneficiaries—the poor and, especially, poor women. Throughout these chapters, we meet residents of Cité Soleil, people who live and, all too frequently, die there. The research, as noted, was conducted in the midst of great political turmoil. Poverty, violence, gender inequality, class prejudices: These hard surface of life dictated that certain interviews had to be conducted clandestinely and put the anthropologist, like the people she sought to understand, in the way of bullets (and insults from above); they also determined the fates of many.

The violence and danger, Maternowska's candid and ongoing assessment of her own place, and her constant shuttling between the worlds of the rich and the poor: These will remind some readers of the work of Carolyn Nordstrom or Nancy Scheper-Hughes. The resulting account will surely be termed partisan. But the idea that all accounts are partial is hardly news, and so knowing that Maternowska's sympathies lie with the poor make this a better and clearer study.

Reproducing Inequities will also be regarded as a specialists' or scholarly book, because Maternowska is accountable to a very large literature in demography, public health, political economy, history, and of course anthropology. She even makes a contribution to the sociology of knowledge. But this is also a book about social theory, if not always explicitly framed in that way. She notes, of course, that "gendered versions of demography" are much needed but they are only the beginning of what would allow us to "make sense of misery," as she puts it. Maternowska was "determined to understand why so few people used the clinic's family planning services, and among those who did visit the clinic why so few returned," and this may seem like a humble enough task, especially if getting an answer takes years. But it was no easy research project, as appears from examining the erroneous interpretations that abound in the clinics, the air-conditioned offices, and in reports and studies. Part of the problem lies in the limitations of the prevalent theories themselves:

> The theories tend to assume a fluid, mutually respected discourse of equality and opportunity between actors and within and among institutions that function at both micro and macro levels. For example, international governments, donor agencies, and their constituents are assumed to be operating with good intentions. Further, the theories dismiss the extent to which large forces—like structural adjustment programs or international aid often directed against national or local will—might affect people's reproductive actions. The ethnographic descriptions of Cité Soleil's households, the family planning center, and the community demonstrate how the introduction and use of family planning in Haiti has long been a contested domain. Placing these local processes within a historical perspective at the national and regional levels demonstrates how the diffusion of information is hardly causal. Interactions—either local or global—prove to be linked to much larger processes infused with social, economic, and political meanings.

This study reminds us that anthropology is just the sort of discipline to unravel such a paradox, as long as our ethnographic and bibliographic research is, like Maternowska's, grounded in a firm understanding of how structure constrains agency. In other words, a political economy alive to social process, including the varied understandings of all of the players, can span the analytic gulf between symbolic or interpretive anthropology and the disciplines that throw into relief the structural determinants of fertility.

I called this a heartbreaking book, and it is. But it is also deeply instructive, revealing not only how Haiti's "demographic destiny" is determined by many forces but also how even well-intentioned efforts to improve health and well-being can come to naught. There is also more than a single ray of hope in reporting, quite unromantically, the courageous struggle of the people of Cité Soleil to survive and, indeed, to improve their lives and those of their children. As Maternowska notes, they are unlikely to read this book (although one young man asked for a copy, along with a dictionary, since he does not read English). *Reproducing Inequities* will, at first blush, win her few friends among those who might read a study published by a university press. But we should all be grateful for Catherine Maternowska's candor, courage, and persistence. This is a big-hearted and reflective book not just about Haiti but also about the vast struggle of poor women, and of their families, to emerge from what Haitians call "indecent poverty." For them, reproductive rights are no nicety of self-realization but are part of the very struggle to survive.

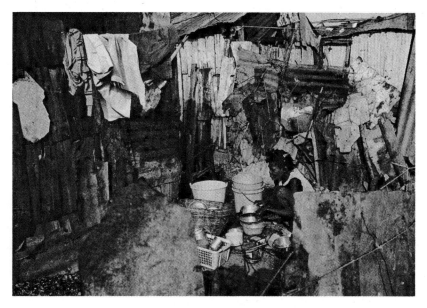

Preparing a meal in a kitchen, Cité Soleil

ACKNOWLEDGMENTS

I am still learning to accept the spontaneous, the strange, and the synchronistic: All the Haitian moments that provoke awe and fear and tears. As I was typing the final paragraph of this book recalling my friend Ernst, I received an email from him. I had not heard from Ernst for over a year. I have known him for nearly fifteen years as an informant, a political organizer, a health care worker, a father, a singer, and in the past few years my bodyguard in the community. The subject line was "surprises" and the text read:

> My friend,
> I am Ernst. I get something for you about CITE SOLEIL. Please, try to
>   write me.
> GOD bless you. Thanks.

It ends up that Ernst, after all these years, is still taking field notes for me. I used to receive crumpled-up notes in the mail that had been dropped in the U.S. postal system by some American traveler to Haiti who met Ernst by chance in Cité Soleil. We have modernized our system of updating each other, with the use of e-mail, but his messages remain fiercely political and always poignant. His report this time was a typically sober detailing of a United Nations peacekeeping raid on innocent civilians in Cité Soleil during July 2005.

There is no reason, really, why a people so repressed by exogenous political forces should have ever trusted such an obvious outsider like me. But they invariably did. I was almost always treated as an honored guest in the country of Haiti, and for that I am profoundly grateful. First and foremost, I extend my deepest gratitude to the people of Cité Soleil. Countless women and men shared their lives—their homes, their food, their time, their stories, their protests, their struggles, and their engaging analysis—with me. When it was too dangerous for me to enter my field site, my closest female companions in Cité Soleil always kept detailed notes for me. When I would return, and after the formalities, they would usually say: "Kati, where is your recorder?" ready to recount events that passed. Many political organizers in Cité Soleil allowed me into their private meetings, shared their notes with me, and always provided keen interpretations of their world. Often, these men and women would go out of their way, some-times missing a day of work and wages, to take me places in the community or throughout the capital of Port-au-Prince. These forays, complete with detailed descriptions, were perfectly articulated for this note-taking anthropologist. In doing this, the people of Cité Soleil merged the realms of critical thought with critical practice and expanded my understanding of just what academic training really is.

Two of my field assistants died: one from HIV/AIDS and the other because he dared to speak out and challenge a political system that was deeply inhumane. In the end, both of these men, and many other acquaintances along the way, were killed by an international order that keeps Haiti trapped and damned by gross inequalities. This book is dedicated to the people of Cité Soleil who have died. And to those who are still "holding on"—*kenbe*—as they say in Creole. You may remain unnamed, but your voices are now recorded as history: a form of power and a right that no one can ever take away from you.

There are also many other Haitians who deserve thanks but must go unnamed because they live and work within the deadly matrix of Haitian politics and position. Making the connections between people and their politics is a major preoccupation of just about everyone in Haiti—from the very poor to the very rich. If one is spotted, even by chance, sitting with, standing near, or simply in the proximity of a well-known journalist, foreigner, political activist, or politi-cian, then one is *enplike*: implicated. To be enplike in the world of international aid and politics, the topic of this book, can be dangerous business in Haiti. Among these people are many Haitian government officials, clinicians, priests, social scientists, agronomists, and activists; I thank all of you for your encourage-ment, your explanations, and your patience. And to the Lambi Fund of Haiti staff and board members, I thank you for taking me into your world; you are lodged in my heart.

When I didn't (or couldn't) stay or sleep in Cité Soleil, I camped in many dif-ferent homes with American, Belgian, French, and Haitian friends—Nicola, Cris, Amy, Sally, John, Alexis, Ira, Daniel, Juny, Jacques, Josette, Loune, Olga, Alain, Frantz, Paul, and many more. These are the people who worried about me when I was out, who fed me when I could not think of food, who comforted me in times of terror, and who soothed me when I had seen too much. These are friends I will never forget.

Through the years, many people offered to read and comment on numerous renditions of this work, including Beverly Bell, Kirsten Moore, Ophelia Dahl, Jane Regan, Julie Meyer, Tally Hustace, Tim Schwartz, Jennnie Smith, and Judith Wingerd. Pierre Minn and Mark Schuller, two graduate students of anthropology in Haiti, were exceptionally helpful and supportive to me, giving critique and raising questions central to the study and practice of development. Talia Inlen-der deserves special thanks for supporting me in the final stages of writing—and lending her intensely political and justice-minded head to the task. Anthony Carter enthusiastically provided a magnificent dose of critique and encouragement. Simon Fass, thank you for your good mind that fueled mine when I needed it most. Photographer of all the illustrations in this book and dear friend Maggie Steber, forever faithful to the Haitian people, thank you for seeing the beauty of Haiti and sharing it with us. Finally, thanks to Deborah Weiss, Patricia Thaxter, and Kim Gilhuly who worked diligently to prepare the text for the press Margaret Case, thank you for your very professional copyediting. All of these advocates of reproductive health have provided knowledge, insight, motivation, and thoughts at different stages of this project, and for that I am grateful.

I have had several mentors who deserve special recognition. My professors at the London School of Economics opened my mind with early critiques of development and set me on a true course. George and Ruth Simmons taught me how demography, reproductive health, and the economy of poverty take shape. Libbett Crandon-Malamud, missed by all who know her, shared the alchemy of critical analysis and compassion. Donald Warwick left a legacy of questioning the politics of population and encouraged me, even through the final months of his life, to keep pushing. Paul Farmer kept faith in the process of my (comparatively) slow inquiry of poverty in Haiti. Finally, I have been deeply inspired by the literary voices of two Latin American authors: Eduardo Galeano for his understanding of history and remembrance, and Gabriel García Márquez for his understanding of love.

I am indebted to my steadfast editor Alan Harwood. Alan worked on this book with an enormous amount of care, determination, and foresight. Alan has been a constant ally; his compassion runs deep. Finally, Alan also carried this book safely to its home at Rutgers University Press and my editor, Adi Hovav. I also thank the anonymous academic critics Alan chose for reviews, all of whom helped this work grow to see the light of day.

In the United States, the Inter-American Foundation and subsequently the Rockefeller Foundation supported the bulk of the fieldwork that led to my dissertation and ultimately this book. Both foundations generously allowed me to ask the questions that many social scientists have overlooked. The findings and conclusions are my own and do not necessarily reflect the perspectives of those agencies.

I am the fortunate child of a large, smart, and politically progressive family. My parents, Elaine and Chet Maternowski, took the responsibility of world citizenship seriously. It was through them—and the teachings of Dorothy Day and the Berrigan brothers, who read poetry in our living room—that I learned the meaning of service and human rights. As parents, they supported my work in Haiti (in spite of their anxiety) and paid for my trips when no one else would. Their view of the world and social justice shines for me still and for this I will be forever thankful.

Last, I am grateful to Alexander, Malcolm, and Caleb—the Cameron boys to whom I am wife or mother and to whom I also dedicate this book. When asked, Malcolm says that his Mama works with "people having babies in Haiti." The truth is that I am able to do this important work because their support and love makes everything possible.

ACRONYMS

APROSIFA	Association pour la Promotion de la Santé Intégrale de la Famille (Association for the Promotion of Comprehensive Family Health)
CCM	Country coordinating mechanism
CDS	Centres pour le Développement et la Santé (Centers for Health and Development)
CHI	Child Health Institute
CIA	Central Intelligence Agency
CMA	critical medical anthropology
CPFO	Centre de Promotion des Femmes Ouvrières (Center for the Promotion of Women Workers)
DHS	Demographic Health Survey
EMMUS	Enquête Mortalité, Morbidité et Utilization des Services (Mortality, Morbidity and Service Utilization Survey)
FHI	Family Health International
FRAPH	Front pour l'Avancement et la Progrès Haïtien (Revolutionary Front for the Advancement and Progress of Haiti)
FWCW	Fourth World Conference on Women
GOH	Government of Haiti
HAS/WHP	Hôpital Albert Schweitzer/Women's Health Program
ICPD	International Conference on Population and Development
INHSAC	Institut Haïtien de Santé Communautaire (Institute for Health and Community Action)
IPPF	International Planned Parenthood Federation
IUD	interuterine device
KODDFF	Komite Ouvriyez pou Defann Dwa Fanm nan Faktori (The Committee of Women Workers to Defend Women Workers' Rights)
KPDSS	Komite pou Devlopman Site Solèy (Committee for Development of Cité Soleil)
MMR	maternal mortality rate
MSPP	Ministére de la Santé Publique de la Population (Minister of Public Health and Population)

NGO	nongovernmental organization
OAS	Organization of American States
OLS	Operasyon Leve Solèy (Operation uplift [Cité] Soleil)
PAHO	Pan American Health Organization
PEF	political economy of fertility
PIH	Partners in Health
PPFA-I	Planned Parenthood Federation of America—International
PVO	private voluntary organization
SOFA	Solidarité Fanm Ayisyen (Solidarity of Haitian Women)
STI	sexually transmitted infection
UNFPA	United Nations Family Planning Association
USAID	United States Agency for International Development
VSN	Volontiers pour la Securité Nationale (Volunteers for National Security)
ZL	Zanmi Lasante (Partners in Health)

Reproducing Inequities

1

Introduction

When Pigs Feasted and People Starved

Menm solèy la nan detrès
(Even the sun is in distress).
–Yolette, Cité Soleil resident, 1993

Route Nationale #1 is Haiti's major thoroughfare. It runs north and south through the capital of Port-au-Prince, directly past the entrance to Cité Soleil, a slum community in the Western Hemisphere's poorest country. Inevitably, traffic backs up for miles on the two-lane road. Exhaust fumes, the incessant noise of huge semis, the suffocating heat, and the smells of squalor make this ride an uncomfortable one. Yet every day, thousands endure it, packed tightly into dilapidated Peugeot station wagons and trucks composed of spare parts. The passengers, many of them residents of Cité Soleil, are displaced peasants going to and from their work within a harsh urban setting, working in construction, selling in the markets, or serving, sunrise to sunset, in the homes of the rich. A market vendor is lucky if her daily wage is US$1, and domestics earn an average of less than US$20 monthly. A single ride along the *route* costs 20 cents, a fare out of reach for the thousands more who must travel by foot in the filthy roadside ditches.

Above this struggling slow tide of humans and vehicles are brightly colored billboards. They advertise things the poor enjoy only in their dreams: Barbancourt Rum, American Airlines weekend getaways to Miami, the ATM machines at the newest Sogebank branch, or the expected opening of Hilton d'Haiti, Haiti's first international hotel chain. Nearly all of this promotion is written in French, the language of the ruling elite, a language most Haitians do not speak. Of Haiti's population, 90 percent speak only Haitian Creole and of those, less than 40 percent can read. For years, though, there was one billboard purportedly designed for poor women. It promoted Minigynon, a low-dose birth-control pill. The graphics depicted a silhouette profile of a woman's head. Her nose was that of a Caucasian, pert and upturned. A tiny pill, held between her delicate fingers, was ready to drop into her expectantly open mouth. The message read: "Minigynon—think of it every day." The message was in French.

Most of the residents who live inside Cité Soleil are landless peasants and their descendants. Accelerating deforestation, unarable land, political repression, and poverty push Haiti's poorest to the capital city in a steady river of migration. Although millions of foreign aid dollars have flooded into Cité Soleil, its residents remain locked in absolute and abject poverty. A lack of infrastructure, including the most basic amenities such as potable water, latrines, and electricity, adds to the generally deplorable conditions. Still, they come to this community *nan chache lavi* (in search of life).

For decades, health surveys completed in this community have made one point clear: There is a strong desire for fewer children (Bernard et al. 1993; Boulos 1985; de Zalduondo et al. 1995; Maternowska 1986; Tafforeau 1989). The women and men of Cité Soleil know far better than any development experts the terrible costs of having and raising children in such wretched conditions.

In the midst of this poor community there was once a family planning center both modern and luxurious by local standards, with running water, occasional electricity, and an imposing wrought iron door to protect the center from vandals. At the height of service provision, the clinic boasted nineteen staff members, an array of modern contraceptives, an accessible location, convenient hours—and yet very few clients.[1] Only 8.5 percent of women and men of reproductive age in the community actually used the clinic facilities; at one point use dropped to 3 percent. Translated into cost-benefit ratios, this meant that international agencies were spending upwards of $50 per client annually in this clinic—half the annual per capita income for most Cité Soleil residents—just to keep a small group of women on birth control.

As a case study, framed in an analysis of gender relations and political economy, this book explores a simple, policy-oriented question: Why don't poor women heed the message of family planning, when smaller families clearly seem in their best interest? Analyzing a decade (1985 to 1995) of family planning policy and practice in Haiti, the focus is on fieldwork carried out in Cité Soleil, Port-au-Prince, between 1991 and 1994. By delving deep into both community and clinic perspectives, this book seeks to explain how residents of Cité Soleil understand family planning and examines the impact of a population program on people's lives.

One day, having interviewed for hours, I persisted in asking one woman what I had asked countless residents over the years: Why did you stop using family planning? Desermite, a former family planning user, gave me her view in starkly political terms. Frustrated by my insistence, she clenched her fists, crossed her wrists and said: *Paske li te esklave m* (because it enslaved me).

How, I wondered, would demographers, traditionally relied upon for interpreting reproductive health data, code "enslavement"? What exactly was the meaning of this enslavement when, in fact, family planning was intended to empower poor women as part of their larger struggles for gender equality? How might this finding and others be interpreted and used by scholars, policy analysts, and development experts who design reproductive health and family planning programs? These responses, writ large, are what this book intends to answer.

Cité Soleil

The community of Cité Soleil is situated on the northern edge of Port-au-Prince in a not-so-contained area of approximately five square kilometers. Open semi-trucks and what were 1970s-style tour buses from the United States transport large numbers of rural peasants from the countryside to the city, in search of life. At the bottom of Haiti's majestic mountains and at the terminus, peasants unload their usually meager belongings and eventually make their way to Cité Soleil. No one really wants to live in Cité Soleil. It is noisy, dirty, politically turbulent, and violent, but it offers cheap housing, the cheapest in all of the capital.

At first glance, visitors to Cité Soleil are impressed by the large avenues and multistory buildings that grace the sides of the central avenue, rue du Soleil. All of these were built and owned primarily by Centres pour le Développement et la Santé (CDS), the nonprofit organization that provides the bulk of health and social services to the community. According to residents, this avenue and most of the other main streets in Cité Soleil were paved to service the many Haitian, U.S., French, Belgian, and German nongovernmental and religious organizations that work in the community. Many residents clearly pointed out, *yo pa t fè sa pou nou* (they didn't make that [avenue] for us). The avenue leads to the center of the community, which is always jammed with carts hauled by men (rather than beasts), traffic jams (packed with sweaty, angry drivers), hundreds of pedestrians, vendors of every ware imaginable, skinny dogs, and pigs. It is very noisy and crowded, and nearly impossible to walk anywhere in the community without pushing or being pushed into people. It is also very hot. During the dry season, the sun beats down so hard that the earth cracks; there is little greenery that can withstand the heat.

The first and only ethnographic map ever made of this community, completed in 1992, divided the community into six large zones: Brooklyn, Linthau, Drouillard, Parc Industriel, Boston, and Centre (Bernard et al. 1993). Within these six zones there are several locales, which in turn divide into *ti katye* or small neighborhoods, named by politically conscious residents for assassinated activists and crowded foreign cities. Off the main road are the innards of this community, twisting and winding through corridors crowded by thousands of tiny shacks situated near dumping areas, open sewers, and putrid-smelling canals. The hot and heavy air that circulates in these corridors shifts in unpredictable directions. Pieces of trash get caught up in these winds, as does the sandy soil. Residents walk shielding their eyes from loose particles known to cause serious eye infections. Space is particularly coveted in the drier areas, just inches above sea level.

During the rainy season, most of the paths blur into muddy tracks and water-soaked ditches: a random sandal, some human excrement, and a gnawed piece of sugar cane litter the mud. When dark clouds hover, valuables are lifted from the floor. Water, replete with feces and garbage during an afternoon or evening rainstorm, can rush up to three feet high inside the homes. One informant, who sold her bed to meet her rent payments, described standing, holding a child in each arm, while filthy water rose thigh-high for several hours in the middle of the night.

From 1991 to 1994, there was no electricity in the community. Economic sanctions and a major dam in disrepair contributed to this crisis—status quo in a country that has never provided a decent infrastructure for the poor. During the same period, the Quartier Général, or army headquarters, the National Palace (also referred to as the "White House"), and selected neighborhoods of the bourgeoisie, far above the slums, were supplied with electricity. Under normal conditions, most residents from Cité Soleil siphon electricity off major power lines to dimly light their homes.

There are some public latrines; however, these are located in the older neighborhoods which had, at one time, better quality housing. One informant told me that over three hundred people living near him shared a row of fourteen latrines. Latrines are either attached to the housing structure or are nearby in the yard, and all are in disrepair. In general, human waste areas are determined by neighborhood consensus and are typically in large dumping areas, or close to the sea. There is no privacy in Cité Soleil, even when defecating.

The community of Cité Soleil houses churches of almost every Christian denomination. There are also at least a dozen *vodou* temples, buried deep within the community. There are many primary and secondary schools, although few people can pay the fees required for books, uniforms, and tuition. CDS, the nonprofit organization that provides health care to the community, manages several schools that teach people skills such as home arts and crafts. There is an old abandoned cinema, in disrepair for over a decade; residents still reminisce about the Bruce Lee movies once shown there.

On the commercial level there are active craftsmen and artisans who "keep shop" on the sides of the large avenues and contribute to a constant din. Street craftsmen make tables, dressers, dining room sets, aluminum cooking pots, baskets, and recycled house products. There are also tire repairmen who work with hand air pumps and homemade tools. Popular lotteries, with names like Celeste Borlette or Solution Borlette, proliferate along the roadsides; residents typically bet on numbers they have seen in their dreams. Community boutiques sell basic necessities such as *malta* (a malt-based thick, sweet, and nutritious drink), Carnation milk, matches, cooking oil, and soap. There are several large outdoor markets where *ti machann-s* (market women) sell produce from rural Haiti or imported plastic products from the United States. Basic necessities like laundry soap or roasted coffee are sold in tiny, single-portion sizes, wrapped tightly into small balls with plastic wrap; residents cannot afford to buy portions larger than what they will immediately use.

One of the community's busiest commercial areas is the *waf* (wharf). Here, small cargo boats with warped masts constructed from skinny tree trunks deliver goods, primarily charcoal and produce, from the countryside to the city. The wharf is large and rickety and always in need of refurbishment. Fishermen sit in groups, repairing their ravaged nets, singing songs of their toils. Women wait patiently as boats approach, hoping to purchase goods such as sugar cane, mangoes, or breadfruit for marketing.

Determining the exact population or composition of people who live in Cité Soleil is difficult, as it is a highly migratory community with strong ties to rural areas. Estimates of the community's population in the mid-1990s were as high as

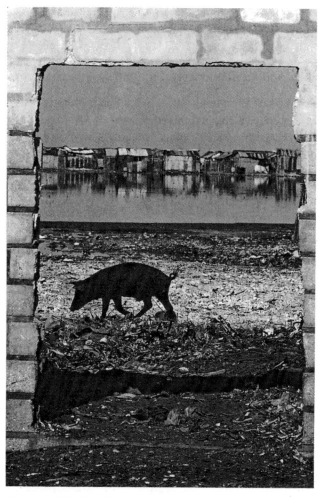

The edge of Cité Soleil

400,000.[2] Most of the residents interviewed for this study were born outside Port-au-Prince and had migrated to the city in search of better economic prospects (cf. Bernard et al. 1993). They came from rural-based farming and marketing families who faced decreasing prospects for production. The majority interviewed also migrated first to neighborhoods with better basic amenities, *pase pòt a pòt* (going from door to door) before establishing residence in Cité Soleil.

Because of the fragile nature of urban survival and still-strong links to the countryside, there is considerable movement in and out of the community. Residents in Cité Soleil usually have several family members in rural areas of Haiti, and they frequently visit these families, often bringing urban goods not available to rural residents. After 1991, many of the new residents were *bòt pipòl* (boat people), migrants who sold their rural land and all of their belongings in hope of finding less suffering in another country. Refugees returned to Haiti by the Immigration and Naturalization Service of the United States Government often joined the ranks of the landless in Cité Soleil upon their return to Haiti.

Pigs and Politics: Survival under the Gun of Terror

Survival has always been arduous in Cité Soleil, made all the worse by political instability—three coups d'état and fifteen changes of government between 1986 and 1994—and violence regularly targeted against the poor. Through a confluence of national political events, in 1986 the people's protest (largely pacifist in nature) brought the infamous thirty-year dictatorship of the Duvalier family to its end, though the structural effects of poverty and politics continue to beset Haiti's poor majority. When "Baby Doc" Duvalier was ousted in 1986, there was an overt change in the political climate, giving voice to the long-silenced poor majority. With the departure of the Duvalier dictatorship, a now burgeoning popular political movement threatened the ruling class structures in Haiti. "The Haitian population set about trying to *dechouke*, or 'uproot,' the traditions of corruption and abuse that had so chronically and so thoroughly permeated the country's power structure" (Smith 2001, 24). Group meetings formerly held in secret and inside dark homes, to protect organizers from military attacks and arrest, now drew hundreds of people in open settings. Popular organizations proliferated and youth movements, many of them instigated in Cité Soleil, began to organize for change. Radio shows once broadcast in French were now transmitted in Haitian Creole and understood by all, thanks to Radyo Solèy. Along with the change of the community's name from Cité Simone (named after Madame Simone Duvalier, the matriarch of the Duvalier family and wife of Papa Doc, Haiti's infamous dictator) to Cité Soleil, the people's popular political movement moved from its underground operations to a clearly public presence within the community.

As with most political organizing, an entire spectrum of parties and views representing the community evolved: Duvalieristes, recycled *tonton makout*-s (armed militia), socialists, anti-imperialists, feminists, and revolutionaries. People organized into diverse forms that included groups, collectives, associations, committees, and federations. There was also considerable spontaneous organizing, some of it determined by women both in Cité Soleil and around the nation. Banging pots and pans and kitchen knives on metal electricity poles and telephone poles, *bat tenèb* (literally "beat back the darkness"), a form of anonymous protest or celebration, was common. Men would join in, hitting a piece of metal or their machetes against poles, fences, or iron gates. The loud clamor signified protest and resistance. During Haiti's prolonged period of political transformation, *bat tenèb* (sometimes originating in Cité Soleil) would spread and bring the entire capital to a standstill with its deafening noise. At the same time, crowds would often take on mass proportions and directions. Once, while in a car in downtown Port-au-Prince, I was caught in what is called a *kouri*. A *kouri*, derived from the Creole verb "to run," was a collective panic or mass hysteria. In a rioting frenzy, crowds would take on directional flows, much like a flock of birds that suddenly decided to change directions. The crowds would move over anything and anyone in their way. In my car with a Haitian friend, we ducked and covered our heads while hundreds of people ran over the car, on the rooftop and across the windshield, shouting in anger. A kouri was typically a mass protest to an announcement on the radio that brought to light some form of injustice.

Following a bloodied attempt at democratic elections in 1987 and then a series of unofficial governments installed under the rule of gun, democratic elections were eventually held in 1990. This was a period when, for the first time in their lives, the residents of Cité Soleil walked peacefully to the polls to vote in their country's first-ever democratic elections. High voter turnout, in urban as well as rural Haiti, led to a landslide victory for the former liberation theology priest Jean-Bertrand Aristide, who was elected president of Haiti on December 16. As a voice for the long-oppressed poor, Aristide's platform was based on redistributing wealth, resources, and power. During his brief tenure he took small steps toward addressing the systemic problems that had long plagued Haiti: lack of a judicial system, the absence of land reform, and an economic system that served the interests of the minority elite for nearly two hundred years. The threat of plans to redress these long-held injustices fueled palpable tension and, seven months later, during September of 1991, a coup d'état ensued.

The era that followed, from 1991 to 1994, the primary backdrop for this study, marked the beginning of one of Haiti's most politically and economically repressive periods. In almost all ways, a study of family planning seemed unimportant during this tragic time, when survival was precarious and Haiti's nascent democracy had collapsed in a siege of extended terror. Further, speaking to foreigners was extremely risky for residents of Cité Soleil. Any contact with journalists—or by extension anthropologists—who might inform the world of Haiti's oppressive regime was dangerous and considered an act of treason.

The coup d'état marked a major transformation in the lives of everyone in this study. Both men and women were affected by the breakdown of civil society in Haiti, which resulted in feelings of helplessness and lack of control. Perpetrators of the coup were determined to erase every last trace of democracy that President Aristide, and the masses that supported him, left behind. The ousted Aristide was supplanted by a military junta and paramilitary thugs who attempted systematically to eviscerate all civic, popular, and professional organizations opposed to its authoritarian rule. The military junta banned meetings throughout Haiti's nine departments. All signs of public protest were swiftly and violently repressed.

Cité Soleil residents were beaten and dragged from their homes for no apparent reason other than having voted in the 1990 democratic elections. Wide-scale, short-term detention served successfully to intimidate and subdue. During detention, vicious beatings were the rule rather than the exception. Almost all arrests were warrantless and illegal (Human Rights Watch/National Coalition for Haitian Refugees 1994). Political repression was particularly vicious in Cité Soleil, since the urban poor in this community were a strong political block for Aristide. Terror ensued; death squads circulated, looking for political activists. By sunset the community was completely silenced: doors shut, windows blocked, even whispers were not tolerated in most households. Rules imposed by the military junta in the community forbade public meetings with three or more people. Residents would recount to me how firing squads rounded up innocent people, murdered them, and forced neighbors to bury the bodies in dumps in and around Cité Soleil. Hungry pigs often discovered bodies stashed behind buildings or buried shallowly in the open trash pits, unearthing evidence of the crimes committed. In response, the paramilitary forces confiscated residents' pigs and then held them ransom for Hg 50 (approximately US$17). During one two-month episode of fieldwork, I observed twenty-two corpses—left on the open dusty boulevards of Cité Soleil with their faces slashed off to impede identification.

Hundreds of people were murdered for having been involved in some form of civic participation or democratic organizing, but more often simply for having voted, or for owning a photo of Aristide (Farmer and Smith 2002). During an emotional point of the fieldwork, when the horror of the ongoing political crisis consumed us all, tears would often surface. One woman held up her hand up to me and in sheer panic said: *Pa kriye Kati, yap touye nou pou sa* (Don't cry Kati, they'll kill us for that). From 1991 to 1994, over 5,000 people were killed in Haiti, 10,000 people were wounded, 40,000 people took to the seas, and 300,000 were displaced countrywide (America's Watch Committee [US] and National Coalition for Haitian Refugees 1993; Farmer 1994). Violent acts against the poor were targeted and deliberate.

To add to the suffering, an economic embargo was imposed on Haiti by the United States with the intent of paralyzing the junta. But the embargo was porous. In 1991, President George Bush exempted U.S. factories in order to protect Haiti's business elite and U.S. capital in Haiti (Farmer 1995). The Clinton administration maintained the same exemptions. Shipments of arms moved over the Dominican border, and gasoline and other "necessities" passed through the ports with impunity. The ruling elite were able to obtain whatever they needed, whenever they needed it. The poor, however, suffered immeasurably. At the time, residents in Cité Soleil felt as if the United States had "sucked" Haiti dry. Between 1990 and 1995, per capita income had decreased by US$100, confirming the country's position as the poorest in the Western Hemisphere. The informal sector, the essence of Haiti's hand-to-mouth economy, turned moribund. Survival was a feat in itself. It was a time when pigs feasted on corpses, but people starved.[3]

Illness imbued everyone's lives. Health indicators, particularly for women, were telling: Maternal mortality in the capital of Port-au-Prince was said to be 1,110/100,000 (CHI cited in UNFPA 1994), making it at the time the highest rate worldwide.[4] Apart from the constant drone of death due to a battery of infectious and waterborne diseases, numerous residents self-diagnosed themselves with *maladi prezidan* (the president's disease). The disease was defined simply as an absence of the people's democracy. It was a time, as a friend from the community put it, when "even the sun was in distress."

Making Sense of Misery

In the face of so much misery, my interview attempts to address reproduction, sexuality, and contraception at times seemed irrelevant. Difficult as it was, I carried on, determined to understand why so few people used the clinic's family-planning services, and among those who did visit the clinic why so few returned. During the three-year period following the coup d'état of September 1991, when most forms of international aid were blocked, contraceptives were exempt from the embargo, and funding for the population sector actually increased. Although the Cité Soleil family-planning center was intermittently closed due to community strife, service provision was more or less continuous.

To my surprise, the importance of these issues was magnified during this repressive era. The collapse of the economy—and the society at large—provided a useful, if not glaringly obvious, stage upon which to examine family planning as part of the United States' aid package. Stripped of almost all of their rights, people generally embraced the interview process. Many of the life histories recorded during fieldwork in Cité Soleil would begin with a resident literally grabbing the microphone from my hand and saying this simple phrase: *Kite mwen bay ou yon ti istwa* (let me tell you a story). Bell (2001:xv) accurately points out that *istwa*, in the Haitian context, refers both to a history and a story as people move "between personal anecdotes and macro political discussion." In the midst of turmoil, issues of reproduction took on heightened meaning, illuminating how inequalities and the structures of poverty affect sexuality and sexual practices (Farmer 1999).

Employing a political economy of fertility (PEF) framework, grounded in an ethnographic critique of a community and its family planning clinic, I show how structures of power in domestic, local, national, and regional terms have determined Haiti's demographic destiny. This book unites three interrelated areas of anthropological inquiry: the contested convergence of anthropology and demography, the politics of gender and reproduction, and the anthropology of development, especially as it relates to technical fixes that evade deeply political questions (Adams 1998).

As a critique of dominant demographic models of fertility (and hence fertility control programs), the book fills a glaring gap in understanding the complexity of reproduction and efforts to control it (cf. Kertzer and Fricke 1997; Greenhalgh 1995). It contributes to a relatively new and critical reassessment of demography by anthropologists and performs a needed service: to help reorient dominant research and scholarly models in the demography of fertility. From its multilevel perspective, the study examines how population policy or "the exercise of power and influence by international actors attempting to achieve a goal" (Finkle and McIntosh 2002) is confounded and, in the case of Haiti, deformed as it filters down to the program level and the demographic targets. The family planning clinic, where policy is practiced, is highlighted as the site where social relations, key to the PEF analysis, are anchored.

Focusing on the politics of gender and reproduction, this book examines the divide between rhetoric and practice in the field of reproductive health. Although contemporary feminist reflections have contributed to rethinking the concepts of gender and power as they relate to demography (Correa 1994; Dixon-Mueller and Germain 2000; Petchesky 2000; Sen and Snow 1994), reproduction (Ginsburg and Rapp 1995), and sexuality (Parker et al. 2000), few scholars have addressed the way these concepts are actually measured and interpreted for application where family planning is practiced. New efforts to measure power and gender as constructs are beginning to take hold (Blanc 2001; Pulerwitz et al. 2000), but these measures tend to be static and often removed from larger structural forces that determine behavior. Viewing gender and power dynamics that affect medicalization, agency, and resistance, I build on Lock and Kaufert's (1998) thesis that women—expanded here to include men—are hardly passive recipients of technological interventions. Through this deeper and more engaged understanding, I show how both women and men relate to reproduction. In the process, I demonstrate how efforts to contain unwanted pregnancies, related high rates of maternal mortality, and the pernicious spread of STIs will remain unsuccessful in the world's poorest countries unless strategies to prevent them are changed to reflect people's realities.

Finally, as a critique of development, this is a study of the multiple meanings of health care, narrowly defined by international agencies, and considerably more broadly defined by political activists who live within the "target" community. Cité Soleil was one of several urban sites in Haiti granted a development assistance contract worth over ten million dollars for general public health improvements. This, however, did not sit well with the poor, most of whom were locked in abject poverty. Residents' reference to the *gwo chabrak-s*—big shots—and their control over the influx of international aid is similar in concept to Adams's (1998) "external profiteering," when international development agencies keep their selected local leaders in business while demonstrating little if any accountability to the poor. The family planning center became symbolic of this profiteering.

The book questions the extent to which public health interventions—in this case family planning—can remain politically neutral in situations of grave social inequality (Adams 1998). The divide between Cité Soleil residents and the Centres pour le Développement et la Santé (CDS), the organization that housed the family planning program—and for many years the United States Agency for International Development's (USAID) favorite nonprofit public health institution—was complex. As a longtime resident in the community, as well as frequent visitor to and observer of the offices of USAID, I was privy to heated political debates about health care delivery from the perspective of the poor as well as that of the powerful. The discourse pits development experts with their seemingly technical and politically neutral approach (Ferguson 1994; Mitchell 2002) against what was one of the most disenfranchised yet politically engaged communities in Haiti. Incorporating the role of development in their analyses, residents uncover the mechanisms by which a population program, formulated without the participation of the community or recognition of their expressed needs, inevitably failed. This account of what happened in Cité Soleil also builds on the work of anthropologists studying health care movements (Morgan 1993; Paley 2001) in politically charged contexts.

Fieldwork Settings and Methods

Collecting data for this research in Haiti was a long and involved process. In 1987, when my first set of taped interviews was stolen (and never returned) by the Haitian military, I quickly realized two important field issues. First, it was clear that being an anthropologist in a politically turbulent community would require great methodological flexibility. Second, to work in these conditions meant practicing "anthropology with one's feet on the ground"—a term Scheper-Hughes (1992, 1997) coined, referring to the "politically grounded practice of fieldwork."

But this was also fieldwork in the midst of social change. Even though democracy in Haiti was short-lived in the early 1990s, people would often tell me, *nou te goute demokrasi* (we tasted democracy), as if to say they would never forget the rights they knew were unalienably theirs. The field context was charged.

Paley (2001) citing Fine (1992) refers to this type of field work as "participatory, activist research," Where knowledge is gathered in the midst of a social change project. This description seems most appropriate for my own fieldwork experiences, even though truly beneficial social change has still not occurred in Cité Soleil or Haiti in general.

In spite of warnings from the American Embassy that dissuaded Americans from traveling to Haiti and curfews imposed by the Haitian government that circumscribed my movement, I had some degree of protection in, and therefore ethnographic access to, this community for several reasons. First, I had volunteered in the Cité Soleil family-planning clinic for many years as a manager, trainer, and facilitator for funders. As a volunteer in 1985, I completed a research study of family planning users and met with over 250 women and their families, so both the clinic staff and clients knew me. Second, in 1987, I implemented the community's first family-planning promoter program and interviewed dozens of women for six available positions. Once the program was under way, I worked closely with the promoters, visiting the neighborhoods and homes of existing and potential clients. I was fairly well accepted by residents. Third, in order to pay for my flights to and stays in Haiti, I worked as a consultant for various health care organizations such as Family Health International (FHI) and the International Planned Parenthood Federation (IPPF), agencies whose programs were financed and directed out of the Port-au-Prince United States Agency for International Development (USAID) office. Few consultants wanted to venture into Cité Soleil; at the time, I was frequently called upon for help in assessing family planning issues there. Although these consultancies gave me little credit among progressives working in Haiti, they provided invaluable insight into the workings of international development aid from the institutional and program perspectives.

Nonetheless, fieldwork was often conducted in fits and starts. From the beginning of the formal data collection there were many political events that made access to the field difficult and, at times, not feasible.[5] In Cité Soleil, shootings, burning barricades or buildings, brutal beatings of innocent people, and demonstrations—either for or against democracy—were commonplace. After the coup d'état in 1991, I no longer felt safe enough to remain in friends' homes for extended stays. Rapes were too common. Typically, I would arrive in Cité Soleil at sunrise and leave at sundown. A network of friends from the community almost always kept tabs on where I was during the day.

My role as an ethnographer was interpreted in different ways. The Belgian nuns who helped provide primary health care to the community asked me to join their order. They would see me in Mass, the community, or at the local hospital, and assumed I had chosen the vocation of working with the poor. I received daily (and appreciated) blessings for my commitment. Some community residents took no interest in my presence and wrote me off as a *blanmanan* (an unknowing foreigner). Others took great interest and considered me a patroness of all causes political and would ask me to photocopy political promotional materials or drive candidates to different neighborhoods to campaign. Some even figured I was either a journalist, because I was always taking notes, or a Central Intelligence Agency (CIA) agent, because I was North American. Most often, the community referred to me by my *ti non* (nickname), Kati Kapot (Cathy Condom), since I was often working in the clinic or in the community side by side with the family planning promoters. This general perception of me as Kati Kapot acknowledged both my alignment with international family planning development projects that were generally criticized by the poor, and emphasized my unique "insider" status that resulted from my regular forays into the community, which set me apart from those who came in and did what the residents referred to as the "business of development."

During the height of repression and as an engaged, "barefoot" anthropologist, I used my protected status to usher foreign journalists into Cité Soleil, a beat they wanted to cover but feared approaching on their own. Equipping reporters with stethoscopes, I posed as a family planning specialist, with a box of condoms in hand, and together we entered people's homes to interview residents about the thick political repression that defined their lives. As a result, many of the residents in Cité Soleil assumed I was also an Organization of American States (OAS) Human Rights observer and would often pull me into their homes and recite to me the horrors they or their neighbors had experienced the night before. The unfortunate truth was that even though Cité Soleil was the site where dead bodies surfaced regularly and violations of the most unimaginable sort were commonplace, no OAS observers were assigned to the community. The murder of an activist whom I knew very well and the ghastly display of his corpse, coupled with massive protest directed at me simply because I was American, propelled me to the nearest phone demanding that a dossier be opened. It was not until I stated fear for my own life that the human rights observers responded to my appeal.

Over time, most of the residents in the neighborhoods that I visited came to accept me as their sounding board. It was during these hours, which blended into days, months, and then years, that my analysis of the politics of health care took shape. The shifting political backdrop to my fieldwork over the decade I spent moving in and out of this community was essential to my understanding of how health and politics interact in Haiti. Like Paley (2001) working in Chile, it is in this context that I saw myself studying political processes *with* the urban poor rather than taking notes and studying them, their actions, beliefs, or behavior.

The formal research protocol was implemented in May of 1991, four months prior to the coup d'état that ousted President Jean Bertrand Aristide. Within days of the coup, hundreds of pro-Aristide supporters, many living in Cité Soleil, were killed during the politically targeted repression that swept the country. At one point, residents of Cité Soleil estimated that over 40 percent of the community's residents had fled into hiding, primarily to the countryside. The family planning center, along with other health facilities, closed intermittently during this period. Because many human rights violations occurred in conjunction with expressions of free speech, meeting with participants in the research, even in clandestine places, put people at great risk. Frequent airport closures and later "lists" with activists' names at the airport made work in Haiti too difficult and dangerous; I commenced preparatory fieldwork in Miami, Florida.

From October 1991, ongoing political violence in Haiti and against the poor only accelerated. Thousands of Haitians sought refuge in the high seas—destined for "any country outside Haiti." Before long, residents of Cité Soleil were populating the Little Haiti community in North Miami, an area that spans fifty blocks and remains home to over 200,000 Haitians. Haitians living in Miami are said to be less Americanized than many Haitians who settle in more northern cities such as New York, Boston, and Montreal, and so the Little Haiti community was a natural field site. Miami-based Haitians are also said to be members of a "younger" immigrant community (the settlement mainly began in the 1980s). As a whole, the members of the community are also poorer and less skilled than immigrants living in more northern communities. I quickly immersed myself in the Little Haiti community by taking a part-time position at the Haitian Refugee Center, where new refugees sought free legal services. Through extensive client and community networking, I located residents of Cité Soleil throughout the greater Dade County area. During this period, I was able to complete the development and pretesting of the community survey instruments and the clinic observation form. I also traveled twice on peace and justice delegations to Guantánamo Bay, Cuba, in search of Cité Soleil residents who had been detained by the U.S. government for leaving Haiti on illegal vessels.[6] Trips between Miami, Cuba, and Haiti clarified the importance of a regional geographical analysis (Hammel 1990).

In anticipation of my return to Haiti, I conducted five household interviews with Cité Soleil residents who had relocated to Miami to escape political violence. Of the five Miami-based participants, there were four women and one male partner. All these subjects had escaped Haiti on boats, passed through the U.S. military facility at Guantánamo Bay for refugee processing, and were classified as "aliens" awaiting judicial proceedings for permanent residency. In addition, I completed five interviews with male political organizers. All of the Miami-based Cité Soleil participants had been in the United States for less than six months. Data were collected based on recall (recording facts and events as if in Haiti), to keep data collected in Miami consistent with that collected in Haiti. Though the initial interviews completed in Miami did not contribute to the overall consistency of the sample, and although the respondents were a select group of individuals (thereby distorting generalizability of the larger community sample in Haiti), this stage of the research offered several advantages that informed the political analysis of this study.

First, people felt freer to talk in Miami without fear of harassment or torture for engaging with a foreigner—a common and punishable crime under the military junta. Political activists from Cité Soleil willingly agreed to be interviewed in their new Miami locales. Second, women interviewed in Miami had typically arrived in the United States without their partners. Most of them viewed this newly found status as liberating. Having tasted life in Miami, people's discussions about their social and political marginalization were opened wide. Last, meeting and reuniting with residents of Cité Soleil reaffirmed an already extensive system of networks that spanned the Atlantic Ocean. This facilitated future introductions to extended families left behind in Haiti and ensured that on returning to Haiti, data collected on recall in Miami (about household composition, reproductive histories, and so on) could be verified. For interviews completed with the Miami-based women, I was also able to cross-check data in the Cité Soleil clinic to verify reproductive and contraceptive histories.

When political upheaval subsided somewhat in Haiti, a return to the field during two extended periods in 1993 and 1994 yielded the remaining data for this study. Prior stays in Haiti, beginning in 1984, enabled me to compare social and economic conditions in the 1990s with those of the 1980s to determine the extent to which events might be altering "normal" survival strategies. What was happening on a political and economic level in Haiti during the early 1990s was clearly part of a steady downward spiral. The fact that over 65 percent of the population of Port-au-Prince lived in absolute poverty was testimony to this crisis (UNDP 1994:165). Instability forced households and individuals constantly to readjust and employ adaptive strategies that Kabeer (1994:158) calls the "crisis-coping capacity of households." How these strategies affected fertility outcomes became central to the research.

In the Cité Soleil community the goal was to understand the complex relationship between residents' health, fertility, and quality of daily life. My methods were standard for participant observer ethnography: semistructured interviews and attendance at rituals and political events. Political activists had gained confidence in me by word of mouth. This led to numerous invitations to grassroots organizing meetings around health care issues that addressed "access" and "need" from the perspectives of the poor.

To uncover varying motivations and behaviors behind high fertility, I divided the community survey sample into subgroups: current contraceptive users, former contraceptive users, and those who had never used contraceptives. All women interviewed were between the ages of 15 and 49 years, the standard public health age range for women in their reproductive years. The universe was defined by the population of adults living within the geographical boundaries of Cité Soleil, as determined by de Zalduondo (1991). Family planning promoters, or women friends in neighborhoods, helped by casually inquiring if women who fulfilled one of the subgroup criteria were able and willing to talk and participate in the study. All people in this study appeared to be genuinely interested in the opportunity to tell their own story, in their own way, to a respectful and sympathetic listener. Securing cooperation was facilitated by the fact that participants were remunerated Hg 150 (approximately US$10) for each interview.

With participants' consent (and that of spouses, when required), I recorded and later transcribed forty-two community-based household interviews (n = 42). In every case where a spouse was present at the time of the interview, the male partner decided whether he or his female partner would be interviewed; the women deferred to their partners' control over this decision. Once the decision was made, all of the men allowed me to complete the interview in total privacy (that is, no men were present when the women were interviewed).

Use of the *mikwòfon* (cassette recorder) was fully embraced among study participants. Journalists in Haiti often record interviews this way and so, for the residents in Cité Soleil, recorders symbolized freedom of speech. Interviews were a rare chance for people to express their concerns—for most it was the first time anyone ever listened to them in such great detail. The majority of scheduled interviews occurred inside the informants' homes. Some informants preferred to be interviewed at a home other than their own in the event that they were being "watched" and suspected of partaking in political activities. In the most extreme case, I conducted an interview twelve kilometers north of Cité Soleil. The interviews were usually completed within an eight-hour time span and typically required two separate visits beyond the initial introduction.

In the family-planning clinic, I examined potential factors contributing to, or detracting from, general quality of care and contraceptive use through observation of doctor-client interactions, staff interviews, and attendance at staff meetings. My presence in and around this clinic since 1985, far longer than that of the majority of staff employed there, was well accepted. The staff always reminded me: *Ou se moun lakay* (you are one of us), indicating a certain degree of familiarity.

Doctor-client interactions, defined as beginning when the client entered the doctor's office and ending when she left, were recorded and later transcribed. Before each observation I secured full consent from clients. To reduce the likelihood of bias, I completed over 250 observations over a four-month period and at two distinct points in time (in 1992 and 1993); providers clearly grew used to having me present. Both providers initially greeted women by name—"Hello, Celeste," for example—when observations first began. By the third or fourth interaction their greetings were entirely absent, which proved to be the norm. Over time, I also interviewed the clinic staff, including the medical director of the clinic, two doctors, two nurses, and six (of nine) family planning promoters, using a loosely structured interview guideline. In addition to regular observation of all nineteen staff members, who were always willing to answer my questions on an informal basis, throughout the study, with permission I also attended and audio-recorded staff meetings.

Finally, I completed ten loosely structured interviews with family-planning professionals (working outside Cité Soleil and within international agencies and the Haitian government's Ministry of Health). Questions were provided in advance to all officials. All of the Haitian officials were happy to meet with me, though two of them asked that I not record their answers. It is significant that all officials from USAID/Haiti refused to be interviewed, even though they too were provided questions beforehand. These officials consistently missed appointments and in the end told me they were not allowed to speak to journalists (or "anyone like a journalist," as I was once abruptly told). Nonetheless, I carefully recorded all of their comments during consultancies, casual conversations, or meetings with USAID personnel over the years, and these field notes provided important—if not key—insights for the analysis. Over the years, I collected many documents, many of them unpublished (such as internal memos from USAID collected during consultancy jobs, data runs, and so on) and, as data sources, these added considerable depth to the analysis from the perspective of international aid and development. I also amassed dozens of trip reports, project summaries, and evaluations written by foreign consultants over the past forty years from the USAID library, and these provided an enhanced understanding of the experts' points of view.

Data collected during the 1990s was later supplemented by several returns to the field between 2001 and 2003. During these visits I interviewed only men from Cité Soleil, enhancing my understanding of the gender system in Haiti. Access to the community, however, was increasingly difficult with every visit. In addition to the familiar warnings from the American Embassy and acquaintances, I was also told during these visits that I would be "eaten alive" by the gangs and *bandi*-s (bandits) that had since taken over the community: The circulation of drugs—in addition to rapes, robbery, and assassinations by armed civilians—were and are common (Haiti Progrès 2002).[7] One resident said I needed authorization from the *chimè*-s (paid street thugs, often with political backing) to enter the community. To accommodate this situation, I hired a field assistant from Cité Soleil to recruit male informants for the study and then interviewed the men at the Holiday Inn, a venue recommended by a local journalist as both safe and centrally located in downtown Port-au-Prince. In 2003, I was able to return to Cité Soleil, but with two Haitian bodyguards from the community by my side. This reentry to the field and subsequent interviews while there helped provide an updated perspective on survival in Cité Soleil.

On Interpretation: Time, Language, and Politics

Time

An important aspect of the data reported in this study is the time frame in which I collected information. My fieldwork was done during a period that spanned a decade, but the bulk of the formal research was conducted between 1991 and 1994, a period I refer to as "the post–coup d'état era," since it spanned a time of extended political instability and repression that followed the violent coup d'état of September 1991 that ousted Haiti's first democratically elected president. I have therefore written in the past tense, recognizing this *moman difisil* (difficult moment), as Haitians often refer to it, as part of Haiti's recent political history. But, like my friends and colleagues Elizabeth McAllister and Jennie Smith, anthropologists who completed their fieldwork in Haiti during approximately the same period, I am deeply troubled that the past tense implies that what happened during that moman difisil is not still going on. The men I interviewed in 2003 acknowledged my discomfort with the political implications of verb tense. When I spoke of the moman difisil nearly everyone looked at me with a puzzled expression, one man even clarified by saying, "Do you mean then or now?"

McAllister (2002:22) notes "use of the 'ethnographic present' has been criticized for creating an ahistorical picture of remote people who are outside of civilized history. Yet a historical tone implies the peoples 'are' history." Like McAllister and Smith, I use both tenses. If the point is historical then I use the historical voice; if the subject or issue is still happening in Haiti I generally use the present—whichever is most appropriate. Although this may be perceived as inconsistent, I believe it is accurate, since it reflects the people's experience from then and now.

Language

All translations are my own unless otherwise noted. I generally provide Haitian Creole phrases, though occasionally I will use French, depending on the setting in which I heard a given quote. The Creole spelling system I use is the phonemic system officially adopted by the Haitian government in 1979. The plural form of a noun in Haitian Creole is noted with *yo* attached to the end. Throughout the text, I have adopted an accepted system for signifying the pluralization of Creole terms within the English text by substituting an "-s" for the Creole *yo* (cf. Smith 2001). For example, *kay* is house, *kay-s* are homes. I follow Creole language quotes and passages exactly as they were recorded.

The value of currency in Haiti is also open to regular "translation," since it fluctuates nearly daily. The Haitian *gourde*, devalued enormously during the economic embargo that followed the coup d'état, has never maintained a steady exchange rate since. Calculations used consistently throughout the text are based on Hg 15 = US$1.00, by which Hg 1 is equivalent to approximately US$.07.[8]

Politics

Politics too, are open to translation and often dangerously so. The politics around population planning assistance in the United States have always been contentious and have been known to change radically with each Republican and

Democratic administration. The United States government's current conservative stance on reproductive health is very narrowly conceived. For example, use of the term "comprehensive reproductive health care" is now discouraged and seen as too liberal (*New York Times* 2003). And government officials who deal with grant applications in the field of family planning have recently advised against using key words such as "sex workers" and "men who sleep with men" (Goode 2003). The implications of these trends (discussed in chapter 6) are threatening international reproductive health programs that work to prevent hundreds of thousands of infant and maternal deaths worldwide. A critique of an internationally funded family-planning program, such as I have written here, could be gravely misconstrued, misquoted, and misused. As such, I feel that it is important to state clearly here that this case study of family-planning in Haiti is in no way intended to support any government's efforts to curtail access to reproductive health—to do this would be to tragically miss the point. Rather, what is provided in this study of family planning politics and practice is a fuller understanding of the many issues that determine fertility and reproduction. The results, if properly interpreted and applied, could lead to improving the provision of essential health care where it is most needed.

All individuals in this study have pseudonyms, as do grassroots organizations in Cité Soleil. I chose to identify all national and international organizations and agencies, however, as they are afforded much more security than that provided to any of the people they intend to serve.

Plan of the Book

As a case study of family planning policy and practice in Cité Soleil, Haiti, this analysis asks two key questions: What influences high fertility and low contraceptive use in this urban community? And, why have international agencies' responses to the problem failed? Both the poor and the powerful have debated the answers to these questions, each group reaching very different conclusions about gender, health care, and politics. Beginning in the homes of women and men in Cité Soleil, the analysis winds through the clinic, the community, and the medical and political institutions that rule in Haiti, and finally into the corridors of power in Washington, D.C. and New York City. Using a political economy of fertility perspective, the book shows how history, gender, power, and culture, all basic constructs to social science, take on dynamic and dramatic meaning in people's lives. The analysis shows how ideas about sexuality and reproduction are fraught with meaning that depends on the social, political, and economic space in which these terms are negotiated and determined. The dialectic that results between reproduction and resistance forms the essence of the study. The object of the study is not the residents of Cité Soleil but rather the political, social, and economic processes they were experiencing, resisting, and helping to generate. Understanding reproduction from this perspective sheds light on previously misguided efforts to reduce fertility, especially in the context of pervasive poverty.

I begin in chapter 2 with an overview of the theoretical renditions of reproduction that have evolved from multiple disciplines, including demography, gender/feminist studies, and medical anthropology. Merging these multidisciplinary perspectives, I introduce the political economy of fertility framework that guides the analysis.

Chapter 3 moves inside the households of Cité Soleil, where a gender analysis shows how fertility control is interwoven in women and men's survival strategies. Strained gender relations and tensions around sexuality impose an enormous burden on poor women, men, and their health. The focus here is on the agency of women *and* men as they negotiate, contest, and defend the often contradictory forces within which their lives are embedded. Documenting the extent to which women's rights are violated, especially inside the secrecy of their homes, helps clarify why so few women feel they can actually use the family planning services available to them. Narratives place high fertility and family outside the realm of the simply biological and squarely inside the social, economic, and political currents that define survival, by gender, in Haiti.

Chapter 4 examines the forces of fertility at work in the family planning clinic itself. Clients' interactions with the larger health care organization demonstrate ways in which dominant voices and institutional forms exercise control over poor women's family planning experiences. In this chapter, I show how clients' resistance to the institutional power exerted over them translates into the widespread refusal of family planning as a reproductive practice.

In chapter 5, interviews with residents and popular grassroots leaders show how reproductive policy and practice in Cité Soleil are not left uncontested. The ethnography presented in this chapter reveals "resistance" as a significant force driving fertility in Cité Soleil. On a collective level, local popular movements organizing for change in the face of economic deprivation and political instability challenge traditional public health efforts as both ineffective and unresponsive to the plight of the poor. The history of specific popular organizing efforts links the failure of the family planning program to a potent combination of national and international policies, which have served to undermine basic health and human rights.

Chapter 6 situates the ethnographic accounts of chapters 3, 4, and 5 within a historically rooted analysis—from slavery to the present—tracing the relationship of fertility and family-planning practice to colonialism, neocolonialism, and the powerful international institutions that resulted from these periods. Within this historical perspective, it becomes clear that local reproductive relations are both constituted by and resistant to more global forms of power (Ginsburg and Rapp 1991). The chapter reviews both historical and currently converging—or, as is often the case, diverging—interests of the Haitian state and international aid institutions. The discourse reveals a faltering health sector, involved in ongoing national and international power struggles about who should determine how health and development strategies are practiced in Haiti. This chapter links family planning to the international arena, revealing a much larger—and often contested—global population discourse. An analysis of Haiti's current political crisis and of the Bush administration's intentions to define and influence reproductive health worldwide is discussed with a similar global perspective.

In chapter 7, I propose suggestions on how Haiti's population sector might be reformed to reflect more equitable solutions to high fertility and the increasing morbidity and mortality associated with poor reproductive health. The chapter focuses specifically on practical, applied solutions for the community, based on a review of four different reproductive health care programs that have met with some success. The book closes with an epilogue providing the reader with an update on Haiti's current political and health care situation.

By exploring the social constructions and institutional practices of family planning and development, this book offers an ethnographic account of changing social, economic, and political conditions and their effect on reproductive health strategies. The analysis contributes to a new, broad reassessment of contemporary thinking in reproductive health and critical medical anthropology, as well as in the field of development studies. It challenges traditional demographic approaches to understanding sexuality, gender, culture, and power within a dynamic international political context.

2

Interpretations of Reproduction

Demography, Anthropology, and the
Political Economy of Fertility

Reality is, of course, always more complex, contradictory, and elusive than
our limited and partial theoretical models and methods allow.

–Nancy Scheper-Hughes, *Demography without Numbers*

Haiti has long presented a population paradox: a stated demand for fewer
children yet persistently high fertility rates and low contraceptive use.[1] National
studies have indicated a high level of awareness of family planning among the
Haitian population, and show that 55 percent of Haitian women did not wish to
have more children, and that this percentage is increasing (EMMUS III 2000;
Guengant and May n.d.). Since the 1970s and 1980s in Latin America and the
Caribbean regions, family-planning programs were touted as a huge success and
overall fertility rates dropped, while that of Haiti stagnated (Bongaarts and
Watkins 1996; Helzner 2002). In fact, between 1977 and 1987, Haiti's fertility
rate edged up—not down—from 4.7 in 1984 to 4.9 in 1992 (Cayemittes and
Chahnazarian 1989; IHS/WFS 1981). At the beginning of the twenty-first century
little has changed. Haiti's total fertility rate today still mirrors what it was over
twenty-five years ago: 4.7 (EMMUS III 2000).[2]

When Haiti's population soared over the seven million mark in the 1990s,
the obvious and most demographically sensible solution was to step up pressure
to make family planning programs more effective. The institutional capacity to
deliver family planning services accommodated. From 1989 to 1992, the United
States Agency for International Development (USAID) population budget grew to
seven times its initial size (USAID 1993). By 1994, family-planning outreach services committed by international donors were valued at US $26.9 million (USAID
1993:2), making per capita population activity expenditure in Haiti twice that of
any other country in the Western Hemisphere.[3] Efforts to improve family planning service delivery included offering a wide selection of modern methods and
the institution of vigorous outreach programs. At the time of fieldwork, women in
Haiti could choose from a greater variety of methods than most American women.

Norplant, for example, was available during country-specific clinical acceptability trials but not yet used in the United States. All of these efforts resulted in a national contraceptive prevalence rate of only 10 percent in the mid-1990s (up 4 percent since 1981), compared to a 60 percent average prevalence rate for the rest of Latin America (Fatahalla 1994).[4]

In this chapter I take on the task of explaining some of the interpretations of reproduction from several disciplinary fields, including demography, economics, history, and anthropology. Building a theoretical framework from which to understand the complexities that have gone into defining Haiti's demographic destiny is a very complicated process. To begin, I show how consultants called on to assist are typically isolated from Haiti's reality from the moment they deplane. This isolation feeds into the tendency to rely primarily on the "well-ordered constructions of the social world" that demographers willingly supply in quantitative format to both the U.S. and Haitian governments and policy makers. Consultants' analyses are often limited to the realm of demography, in part because "demography has always been close to the seat of power, employed in the study and execution of policy" (Hammel and Friou 1997:176; cf. Kreager 2004). To provide context to how this power works, I review traditional, expanded, and then gendered versions of demography that have evolved over the decades. In the sections that follow I review anthropology's contribution to understanding population trends, and the rise of medical anthropology and its affiliation with studies of political economy. Finally, merging all these perspectives, I introduce the political economy of fertility as the framework that guides this study.

The View from Above: Demography and Development in Haiti

Foreign consultants and other population experts have frequented Haiti for over forty years now, determined to solve its peculiar population paradox. The nexus of this consultant activity is at the USAID Health, Population, and Nutrition office. To get to the "mission," as it is often called by local expatriates, usually one drives through what seems like all of humanity personified, downtown Port-au-Prince.

The capital of Port-au-Prince, designed to accommodate approximately 150,000 people, was once the metro center for the Pearl of the Antilles—a lovely seaside city, lined with green parks, bustling with commerce, and boasting a coastal view replete with palm trees that paralleled the best in all of the Caribbean. Today, it is estimated that somewhere between 750,000 and 1.5 million people are crammed onto Haiti's once-clean boulevards. Walking these streets is hazardous, as sidewalks are barely discernable from gutters. Someone is selling something from almost every corner. Exhaust fumes, rancid smells, and heat predominate. Everything is made filthy by the lack of public services. Piles of garbage rot along all the streets. Competition for a space to beg on the streets is

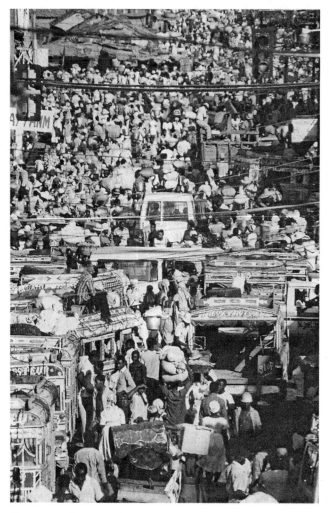

Downtown, Port-au-prince

furious: Legless indigents roll on pieces of plywood fashioned with wheels and plead for coins, while older children will maim younger newcomers to defend their turf. Air-conditioned SUV owners lock down their doors and keep cool within their darkly tinted vehicles. Traffic is helter-skelter; occasionally a police-man will try to direct the congestion that keeps traffic at a near standstill. Street-lights, always out of repair, dangle from shredded cables. *Tap tap-s*, the nation's hand-painted, brightly decorated popular mode of public transportation (these are actually pickup trucks with an extended open-air cab in the back), crowd the streets along with used yellow school buses that were imported to Haiti to "solve" the transportation crisis. I once saw a taxi cab with its missing windshield replaced by cardboard, except for a small rectangular hole just big enough to let the driver inside see where he was heading.

Just south of this epicenter of activity are the USAID offices, situated on Harry Truman Boulevard. A huge fortresslike wall keeps government employees safely sealed in, and out of sight. Those entering must undergo perfunctory car searches as a preliminary security check. The offices are housed in what was once the Beau Rivage, a lovely tropical hotel owned by an Italian and French couple; visitors cross a tiny footbridge (with koi swimming below) to enter into the icy cold air-conditioned interior of the agency. Another series of sensors keep unwanted visitors from entering the facility. Phone calls are made to announce visitors; an official USAID representative escorts everyone to their assigned destination. Lovely tropical plants abound, festive Haitian art hangs everywhere, and there are dozens of corridors that lead in every direction to the various branches of the agency.

It is within the Health, Population, and Nutrition Division that consultants are briefed and provided documents that describe the population paradox. Most meetings are held within this building. Occasionally consultants will conduct field visits, but not always. The in-country advisor to International Planned Parenthood Federation (IPPF), for example, lived in Haiti for nearly five years before he ever entered the site that housed a former Cité Soleil family planning clinic funded by the agency—and that was after persistent urging on my part. Days before his departure from Haiti he managed to visit the community. His comment upon arriving in the dark clinic, lacking ventilation and crammed full of clients: "*C'est coincée ici!*"(It's crowded in here!). The reluctance to visit the field is not uncommon, so in fact many evaluations of and research on family planning programs are explicitly removed from reality.

Many of the major discussions about family planning programs and certainly the laptop report analysis and writing by U.S. consultants takes place up the hill from the USAID offices at the Montana Hotel, a true Caribbean delight. Breezes sweep through the hotel, with its grand lobby made of imported marble. The Montana is always buzzing. Foreign journalists like this hotel; there is electricity and a DSL line, and the telephones work. The hotel hosts an array of events ranging from a lay workers' Episcopal Church conference to swank cocktail parties for members of the Organization of American States. Magical little rocky coves with water fountains and semiprivate areas defined by flowering tropical foliage harbor groups of hushed Haitian elites, usually men dressed in suits, discussing their government, the U.S. government, or both. Outside, huge patios serving international cuisines surround a grand pool complete with a bar that serves the hotel's famous rum punch. From here, there is a sweeping panorama of Port-au-Prince: Carrefour, a sprawling zone that leads to Haiti's southern corridor, the National Palace, the city's main cemetery downtown, and then Cité Soleil, a parched slab of land jutting out into the Bay of Port-au-Prince. Haiti is beautiful from here. This is the view from above.

This view from above is complemented by demographers' "analyses [of] population problems through sets of 'fixed' social categories, which have to stand proxy for what are known to be much more dynamic relationships and processes" (Szreter et al. 2004:223). These quantitative interpretations provide a statistical portrait of this struggling island nation and are used by development officials to justify family planning interventions. Yet, standing as a hemispheric outlier, Haiti continues to defy most standard demographic trends. While the Western Hemisphere region as a whole has made exceptional progress in reducing high fertility, largely attributed to strong family planning program commitment (Helzner 2002), Haiti has not. A recent analysis by Population Action International (PAI 2001) corroborates this in a statistically sharp way, ranking ninety one developing and forty two developed countries (representing 95 percent of the world's population) in one of five sexual and reproductive health risk categories. The study shows that all nineteen countries in the very high-risk category are in Africa, except for Afghanistan and Haiti.[5]

Local and foreign demographers and development consultants have long recognized the country's burgeoning population as bordering on disaster. Warnings of impending growth were first published in the late 1950s, when Haiti's population was three million (Moral 1961). Demographers (May et al. 1991b) divide the history of Haiti's family planning programs into three distinct phases: "A Promising Start" (1967–1982), "The Decline and Disintegration" (1982–1987), and "Toward Recovery" (1987–1991). My own archival research suggests that May et al. overlooked the actual date of initial demographic studies in Haiti. Initiatives were under way beginning with the country's first census in conjunction with the U.S. Marine Corps in 1932 (during a nineteen-year long occupation) and then later in the 1950 census.

"A Promising Start" was ushered in with references to Haiti's population problem and dire warnings of the effects of rural overpopulation. With results culled largely from the 1950s census, Haitian demographers proposed reforestation, road building, open access to markets for farmers, land tenure reforms, and a basic change in the parasitic elite-dominated crop marketing system, all as the means of heading off a "Malthusian" situation. Haitian professionals had a significant role in the initial evolution of family planning practice—an activity they considered essential to the broad definition of community health. In the early 1960s, oral contraceptive research done in tandem with the infamous Puerto Rican trials was already completed, confirming the method to be both safe and effective (Pincus et al. 1959). By the mid-1960s, seventeen facilities were supplying family planning services as part of larger primary and community-based healthcare activities. In 1964, Haitian leaders were part of an international trend that was acknowledging the problems of overpopulation. These programs offered oral contraceptives and later interuterine devices (IUDs), and officials were pleased with the rapid takeoff. The then President-for-Life François "Papa Doc" Duvalier waffled at first, though by 1969 he endorsed the concept of family planning and decided to control all initiatives in the area. During this period, however, the Haitian government was threatened by increasing "foreign control" over the process.

The presence of international agencies ushered in a new era of programming in Haiti. By the late 1960s, family planning's supply-centered activism took hold with great fervor as contraceptives flowed into Haiti, supplying selected clinics throughout the country. By 1967, pro-family planning activism, underwritten by the congressional earmarking of U.S. government funds for international population activities, accompanied an even more zealous focus on supplying contraceptive services (Green 1993). Attempts to incorporate truly Haitian strategies, those that integrated family planning services into other community-based activities, were stymied as they were reformulated, redirected, and redetermined by external funding sources (Bordes and Couture 1978). By the 1970s, the locus of family planning control shifted into the hands of large international foreign aid agencies such as the Pan American Health Organization (then still part of the World Health Organization), USAID, the Pathfinder Fund, the Population Council, and the International Planned Parenthood Federation. The family planning "industry," as Demeny (1988) named it, was up, running, and gaining remarkable speed in Haiti.

What was happening in Haiti was part of a larger international trend that began in the 1960s, whereby population activities moved into a separate sector of development (Szreter 1993). The mandate behind foreign assistance bifurcated health so that primary health care and family planning became two separate sectors—no exceptions were made. Under pressure from USAID, all official public health endeavors in Haiti, from 1971 onward, had separate population components. The parliament approved the revision of the Department of Public Health and Population, and it was subsequently made into law August 26, 1971, with article twenty-six creating a Division of Family Hygiene. Article thirty-nine clearly defined the responsibilities of the division as "supervision and coordination of all activities, public and private, concerned with child health, *including family planning*, in the territory of the Republic" (author's emphasis, Bordes and Couture 1978:165).

The separation of family planning from health care and other development initiatives did not go uncontested. When the link between socioeconomic development and fertility was omitted from U.S. policy, it marked a profound trend worldwide. In March 1971, when preparations for increased international family planning funding were in the final stages, the government of Haiti's director general of the health department, Dr. Lauvinski Faucher, issued a communiqué that forbade "the functioning of all centers, clinics, offices, and others involved in family planning services"(Bordes and Couture 1978:152). Although this appeared on the surface to be a move against the provision of family planning, in fact the communiqué foreshadowed what would be an issue of ongoing concern: restraining the activities of the uncontrolled proliferation of groups, namely private-voluntary organizations, working without coordination with the Haitian government. Eventually the ban was lifted, and by 1976 the declaration of a public health policy within Haiti's first national health plan separated family planning as a distinct component. This declaration was in turn backed by an impressive commitment of international funds. The implications of this policy change in Haiti are central to this study (chapter 6).

By the second demographic period, "The Decline and Disintegration," the government of Haiti (GOH) showed less enthusiasm in its support of the national family planning program, partly because their control of this sector was largely usurped by international funding agencies. In 1987, a large-scale national survey indicated a drop in contraceptive prevalence (EMMUS I 1987). Analysts were quick to point to Haitians as having lost momentum. Although Haitians indeed may have lost momentum, in interviews on the subject they indicate that their momentum was tied up in continued political power struggles with largely Western development rhetoric and control.

In February 1986, the Duvalier family was ousted from Haiti, and political instability and economic difficulties ensued. Family planning program activities were at a lull around the country. For example, during fieldwork in the summer of 1987, the family planning center in Cité Soleil was closed two weeks out of every month due to national strikes and state-imposed curfews. Soon after the departure of "Baby Doc" Duvalier, the U.S.-funded private sector played an increasingly important and prominent role in family planning provision. On December 23, 1987, following what USAID called "the abortive [presidential] elections of 1987," the U.S. government discontinued assistance to the GOH and the public-sector Family Planning Outreach Project was terminated (USAID 1993). All USAID assistance was rechanneled through the private nonprofit and for-profit sectors.

In the years following Jean-Claude Duvalier's fall and during the period that demographers have called "Toward Recovery," 1987–1991, two elements contributed to an apparent—though very slight—upturn in family planning activities. First, analysts point to a noncommercial sector program launched in 1987 with the financial assistance of USAID. While this project incorporated public-sector clinics (that is, those staffed and managed through the Haitian government's Ministry of Health), the familiar pattern of U.S.-imposed control over project content remained. Second, the various governments of Haiti since 1986—only the Aristide government elected democratically and all of them with puppet ministries—showed variable interest in population and family planning activities. Clinical acceptability trials for Norplant, initiated through U.S. interests, led to heavy promotion of the method. Funding continued to flood the sector; by 1988 the family planning sector alone was valued at thirteen and a half million dollars.

Improvements during and beyond the so-called "recovery" period of the population sector, backed by heavy foreign investment, led to a contraceptive prevalence increase of only 4 percent over an eight-year period (1988–1995). Although international experts and select officials applauded this gain, it was scant by any demographic measure.[6] Lant Pritchett, an economist who studies demography, put it bluntly: "Where contraceptive prevalence is having an effect it really has an effect and this is clearly not the case in Haiti" (personal communication 1995).

By Western Hemisphere standards, Haiti's progress in family planning is at best very poor. Even if contraceptive prevalence climbed approximately 4 percent during the period under study, it did not affect overall fertility rates, and there has been a general failure to achieve better health and quality of life for women, men, and children.[7] Three decades since the population control sector's inception, the institutions that usurped control of the public sector—including USAID, IPPF, the Population Council, and several others—were still actively working in Haiti in the 1990s.[8] A great proportion of their work was spent determining why family planning efforts have failed so markedly but, ultimately, their efforts to effect change have been minimal (Augustin and Gay 1991; Burton 1989; CARE-International 1993).

Although demographic statistics have yielded some information related to why fertility remains high and contraceptive use so low, demography's proposed solution to Haiti's population problem, namely, focusing on increasing contraceptive prevalence rates while lowering fertility and birth rates, is cast in unduly narrow terms. A brief review of the guiding theories of demography and anthropology helps explain why the traditional demographic response has failed and how the theoretical strength of the political economy of fertility framework, which builds on expanded notions of both disciplines, can provide a powerful guide for understanding and addressing family planning practices in Haiti.

Demography's Diagnosis

In Haiti and elsewhere, large-scale demographic survey results continue to guide most population policy and programming. Use of these surveys as a means of measuring population change was first introduced in 1941, based on the concern around fertility decline in the United States. Postwar declines in mortality (resulting in part from the introduction of public health programs worldwide) soon shifted part of the U.S. focus overseas. Presser (1997:301) remarks, "A central task of American demographers became convincing third world leaders that population control was both needed and possible." The first large-scale surveys introduced overseas were the Knowledge, Attitude, and Behavior surveys, with followed soon after by the World Fertility surveys.[9] But concerns about population growth and its effect on society date considerably further back, to Malthus's apocalyptic warnings in 1798 of overcrowding and starvation. Efforts to predict macro population trends—and to explain the causes of these patterns—have consumed demographers, economists, and other social scientists since the early part of the last century.

For decades now, demographers have relied largely on the classic demographic transition theory to inform their understanding of population trends. The theory first introduced by Notestein (1953) outlines three stages through which a country's population is likely to pass: initial high fertility and high mortality, followed by high fertility and low mortality, and finally into low mortality and low fertility. Although various worldwide trends have been documented at one stage or another, not all countries have actually transitioned. Divergent patterns of fertility decline worldwide, evidenced by large-scale demographic surveys in the 1970s and early 1980s, indicated the increasingly poor predictive power of the theory. The European-based patterns on which the original theory was based clearly have little to do with a great number of relentlessly impoverished countries caught in varying stages of development. Countries like Haiti, snagged in the early stages of the transition, have failed to move to a low fertility stage in spite of heavy family planning inputs.

Numerous demographers have sought to explain these differing patterns of transition; two of the more recent efforts encompass multiple levels of analysis as well as social, political, and economic variables. Bongaarts and Watkins (1996) explain why, as in Haiti, a 50 percent drop in infant mortality nationwide, from 1960–1992, signaled the first trigger of a typical demographic transition without a corresponding dramatic drop in fertility rates (UNICEF 1994b). In their impressive study to discern variability in patterns of decline in sixty nine developing countries over time, the authors propose that the pace of fertility decline is not necessarily related to the pace of development, but rather to the level of development when the transition began.

This theory assumes that countries with stalled demographic transitions can expect to enter a transition in the next few decades, spurred not by any improved development indicators per se but by a series of social interactions at the personal, national, and global levels. Building on the concept of information diffusion, the authors elaborate on the importance of "a process by which innovation spreads among regions, social groups, or individuals, often apparently independently of social and economic circumstances" (1996:656).[10] Bongaarts and Watkins argue that key elements to the transition are the exchange of information and ideas (such as information about contraception), the evaluation of their meaning in a given context (the potential acknowledgment that fewer children might make life easier), and social influence (a subsequent trend that ultimately sparks widespread use of contraception). Social interaction, then, is seen as a force that triggers changes in population dynamics, notably fertility behaviors. Further, the authors imply that a domino effect will occur once a few countries in a given region enter the transition to low fertility levels, with other countries following.

Soon after Bongaarts and Watkins's model, Caldwell (1997) proposed a need for a unifying theory, a "global fertility transition," uniting the first, Western (European) fertility decline with the second, contemporary third-world decline.

Caldwell advocated the importance of long-term economic and demographic trends along with ideas, ideologies, legitimation, and assistance in access to contraceptives. He argues that social interactions at the personal and community level are less important than global interactions. Caldwell cites Bangladesh's well-known success in family planning, following what was once a worst-case scenario replete with devastating poverty, significant religious and gender barriers, and a stalled transition. Bangladesh serves, then, as an example of a "conversion of government and national elites, taking on the task of commitment to a national family planning program" (1997:810).

Both of these neotransitional models move beyond the original population theorists and are appropriately linked not only to contraceptive technology transfers from North to South, but equally to other directional flows among and between local, national, and international channels. Bringing social and even political processes into demography breaks the narrow scope of demography as a science determined to quantify.

And yet these models remain distinctly removed from a jagged reality that dominates in the world's poorest countries. The theories tend to assume a fluid, mutually respected discourse of equality and opportunity between actors within and among institutions that function at both micro and macro levels. For example, international governments, donor agencies, and their constituents are assumed to be operating with good intentions. Further, the theories dismiss the extent to which larger forces—like structural adjustment programs or international aid often directed against national or local will—might affect people's reproductive actions. The ethnographic descriptions of Cité Soleil's households, the family planning center, and the community demonstrate how the introduction and use of family planning in Haiti has long been a contested domain. Placing these local processes within a historical perspective at the national and regional levels demonstrates how the diffusion of information is hardly causal. Interactions— either local or global—prove to be linked to much larger processes infused with social, economic, and political meanings.

Elaborating on Demography

Although emerging demographic and economic theories may shed some light on differing patterns of population decline, overall the micro processes that ultimately affect reproductive behavior are not well understood. This has stymied effective population programming and practice in "high risk" countries, since population policy is almost always based on large-scale demographic trends. The basic limitation of demographic analysis has been its tendency toward the macro perspective (by isolating variables and generalizing across a social situation) rather than the comprehension of micro processes. Some demographers, however, have sought to broaden demography's scope to include consideration of micro-level factors alongside macro-level determinants.

In a collection of essays entitled *Diffusion Processes and Fertility Transition*, Carter (2001) takes a broader view of fertility change and diffusion while maintaining the link to social processes and cultural variation. His critique is particularly fitting for this analysis in Cité Soleil, which explains, in deeply complicated ways, through local, national, and regional settings, that family planning cannot be reduced to a notion or technology sent as a form of development assistance. Carter notes, "The ubiquity of diffusion conceived of as cultural flow is not simply a reflex of the rapidity with which new knowledge is generated by the scientific establishment of the rich nations at the core of the global economy and transmitted to all the nooks and crannies of the periphery by global institutions devoted to development and technological transfer. Novelty is generated continuously throughout the global system, including in its more or less peripheral nooks and crannies" (2001:167).

It is from the "nooks and crannies" within Cité Soleil that local reactions to family planning are contested and negotiated (though rarely accommodated). Although reasons for rejecting family planning are explored throughout this book—in different settings and over time—the actual diffusion of contraceptive information and meaning, as Bongaarts and Watkins propose, is infinitely more complicated than simply an exchange of information and social interaction alone. Social interactions in the Haitian setting are replete with meaning as women and men, clients and providers, and even Haitian professionals and U.S. development experts' struggles are placed within the larger social structure. These interactions, Carter argues, are all "culturally defined and immensely variable" (2001:167).

In addition to Carter, other demographers have argued that traditional demographic theory should be expanded upon, given the evidence that "off-the-shelf" population policies have failed to resolve high fertility trends in the same way around the world (Cain 1981, Kreager 1982; Lesthaeghe 1980; McNicoll 1978, 1983, 1993a, 1993b). In arguing for an expanded demography, McNicoll (1978:690) notes that "the complexities that go into determining how a population goes about recruiting its next generation are collapsed into a total fertility rate, as if both policy makers and parents were or should be concerned overwhelmingly with this one outcome."

Providing an alternative to these theoretical models, Kreager (1982) examines how social processes determine demographic preferences (as well as differences) in rural pastoral societies from Eastern and Central Africa. Kreager argues that deeper understandings of the social institutions and strategies that affect the social control of sexuality and fertility are key to fully understanding the variation of demographic patterns. He notes, "if models of demographic behavior are to be made more accurate, they will need to follow more closely the cultural conventions and categories that order peoples' own understanding and use of these institutions" (1982:237).

McNicoll offers yet another alternative theoretical approach to expanding demography's scope with his "institutional determinants" theory, cited by anthropologists for its comprehensiveness (see Greenhalgh 1995; Kertzer and Fricke 1997). The "institutional determinants" theory moves toward an understanding of both macro and micro dynamics, situating them within larger structures such as class, lineage, and political and administrative institutions. McNicoll (1993b:5) defines institutions as "clusters of behavioral rules governing human actions and relationships in recurrent situations . . . generating society's distinctive patterns of social organization." The theory embraces individual behavior and the way in which institutions are affected by local, economic, and historical forces attending to cultural specificity.

McNicoll's institutional approach harkens to the original theorists of institutional behavior, such as C. Wright Mills and John Rex, who cautioned that "institutions may be looked upon not as an affair of participation in consciously shared common purposes, but as forms imposed and maintained by a ruling elite for their purposes" (Firth 1964:22). In the world's poorest countries (where fertility tends to be highest) institutions are created, maintained, and often reinforced by the elite, or by those with access to forms of power. Whereas dimensions of power may be tacit in McNicoll's institutional perspective, they are not central to the analysis. Notably, the role of the individual actor or agency—vis-à-vis power—is somewhat buried in these theoretical frameworks.[11]

Gender Studies and Demography

In addition to the contributions of social interaction and institutional determinants theory to the field of demography, feminist scholars have sought to expand demography to include considerations of gender. Until recently, gender had been largely ignored by demographers and policy makers, since it is difficult to measure and interpret (see: Dixon-Mueller 1993; Mason 1987; Mason and Taj 1986; Oppong 1983). Historically, as a discipline, demography viewed demographic outcomes as dependent variables and gender as an independent variable (Presser 1997; Watkins 1993). There have been some advances in the field, documented in Haiti's most recent Demographic and Health Survey 2000, with an impressive addition of gender-related measures that attempt to capture women's status through measures of couples' communication, opinions on gender roles, economic autonomy, and domestic violence. Although this marks a notable advance from previous demographic surveys, these measures provide only a snapshot of the problem and fail to uncover reasons behind women's status, what might change this status, and how this information might be incorporated into family planning programs.

The feminist movement during the 1980s and 1990s had as its basic goal women's control over their fertility and sexuality. Folbre's (1983) work on the historical decline of fertility with a focus on gender relations was, at the time, a lone voice in demography circles. Her focus on the changing power relations within the family, including emerging patriarchal inequalities between men and women under capitalism, moved the gendered perspective more squarely into demography. Adding strength to the argument, Handwerker (1989), armed with individual and societal-level data from Barbados, made similar links between gender and demography, critiquing the tenets of standard demographic third world fertility decline and family planning policy. He argues that fertility transitions will occur when women's power relationships within the family, and notably with men, change. Handwerker's focus on women's access to power and resources concludes that providing women with education, employment, and family planning is key to modernization.

The 1980s marked a new era that combined the strength of both academics and advocacy with coalitions of feminist scholars and activists, many from Southern countries—including Latin America, the Caribbean, Africa, and Asia—who entered debates about population growth and fertility rates. Feminists argued that the reproductive health sector's preoccupation with fertility reduction, especially programs that were target-driven—or heavy-handed—were resulting in numerous violations of women's rights (Petchesky 1998). Academics, practitioners, and activists in the field pushed to place reproductive health within a basic human rights framework. Their demands included the provision of safe, effective methods of contraception and abortion, improved conditions for childbearing, sexuality free from violence and disease, income-generating opportunities, and food security. The basis of these demands was simple: dignity and respect for women as clients of services and as human beings (Petchesky 1998).

Haitian women joined these debates in 1986, a year marked by the departure of the oppressive Duvalier regime. In the isolated mountain town of Hinche, four hours by deteriorating roads from the capital, politically active, organized Haitian women were echoing similar sentiments.

> We need to understand the struggle that women in other countries are leading for their rights. We need to know what is happening not only in our own country but also in the Caribbean and in Latin America. These women are living in small nations which are poor like our own, and which the big countries are sucking dry. We must learn from the good work of women in countries around us. We do not need any prepared recipe— even if it comes from the house of Uncle [Sam]—to come tell us what is good for us. We are not ignorant: we can think for ourselves. We know what we need and don't need. (Caritas of Haiti 1986:1)[12]

By the 1990s, analysis devoted to the social control of reproduction (Sen and Snow 1994), population and reproductive rights (Correa 1994), and population policies (Sen, Germain, and Chen 1994) added to the discussion of the notion linking women's bodies with social, political, and economic rights and the conditions required to achieve gender-based justice (Batliwala 1994; Correa and Petchesky 1994). Even within this new framework, however, some feminist demographers were still calling for quantitative and positivistic data in order to make the links between gender and demographic change (Mason 1997). The construction of sexuality in this approach left little room for family planning clients' own interpretations about their sexual lives and the power relationships that constitute gender relations, provider-patient relations, and individuals' situations within larger communities. Demographic assumptions that narrowly defined women's needs expanded during the decade, though the discipline remains limited in theory and practice.

The product of decades of feminist groundwork appeared on an international stage at the International Conference on Population and Development (ICPD) in Cairo in 1994 and again at the Fourth World Conference on Women (FWCW) in Beijing in 1995. Pressure to embrace reproductive health from a human rights perspective helped move narrow family planning discourse to a broader platform that included women's health and empowerment issues, linking reproductive and sexual rights to women's rights (Hartmann 1995; Petchesky 1998). Although ICPD was considered a benchmark in the history of reproductive health consensus making, setting admirable reproductive health goals, what has happened on the ground since 1994 lags far behind. Petchesky (1998:4) puts it bluntly: "Having achieved considerable success at the level of theoretical visions and United Nations rhetoric, feminist activists in all the world's regions now face the problems of turning reproductive and sexual rights into concrete realities in women's everyday lives."

The feminist agenda, promoting women's reproductive health as more inclusive than simply family planning, has rhetorically made huge inroads (Wang and Pillai 2001; Zierler and Krieger 1998). However, in Haiti there has been little impact on local discourse or practice. Haitian representatives were present at the conference in Cairo and signed, along with 178 other countries, the declaration establishing guidelines for population and reproductive health programs. Five years later, during a visit to Haiti, I inquired of USAID's senior health and population policy advisor if and how the guidelines were being implemented. In e-mail correspondence several weeks later, the advisor noted that the Haitian government liaison responded in two separate but symbolically related points: "To our knowledge, there is no official mechanism [in place] to implement the Cairo conference. The official *Revue du Sénat de la République* argued in 1998 for the formulation and implementation of a population policy, but without success" (My translation from French, personal correspondence, Coyne 1999).

Anthropology and Reproduction

Along with demography and gender studies, anthropology has long been involved in recording reproductive behavior. However, the study of reproduction was not, until recently, central to the field (Ginsburg and Rapp 1991). Browner and Sargent

(1996) trace the study of reproduction and fertility, as well as interest in demographic issues, to the 1930s with Malinowski's work on the reproductive health practices among the Trobriand Islanders and later in the 1940s with Montagau's study of the concepts of conception and fetal development among the Australian aboriginals. Szreter et al. (2004:2) also provide an elaborate review of historical anthropological demography, noting how "demography's 'vital events' commonly are celebrated by anthropology's 'rites de passage.'"

Through the 1960s, most reproductive anthropology work focused on beliefs or values surrounding reproductive behaviors. By the end of the 1960s, notably with Ehrlich's publication of *The Population Bomb* in 1968, a growing number of fertility studies took more anthropological perspectives (see, for example, Nag 1975; and Polgar 1971, 1972). Abernathy (n.d.) recalls a comprehensive health care project in Khanna, India, that showed the futility of attempting to change family size preferences with even the most inclusive health care programs (Wyon and Gordon 1971). Mamdani carefully analyzed the family planning component of Wyon and Gordon's project in Manipur and produced *The Myth of Population Control* (1972), which served as one of the earliest critiques of family planning. The critique documents local indifference to and failure of a family planning experiment. For six years, Wyon's group provided a whole village with education, nutritional supplements, public health, and direct medical care. Eventually everyone knew about contraception, villagers had positive attitudes toward the health care providers and family planning, and infant mortality had fallen way down. But the fertility rate stayed high (Wyon and Gordon 1971).

Mamdani's study was important for being among the first to reveal both social and economic rationales behind reproductive decisions in poor families. In this village-level study, the program's failure was attributed not to villagers' misunderstandings or ignorance (even though project personnel claimed this was the problem) but rather to economic, and largely agricultural, conditions that worked against small families.

Nag and Kak (1984:676) returned to Manipur twelve years later to collect survey data and found contraceptive prevalence in Manipur had increased to 50 percent. Drawing on their own data as well as Mamdani's socioeconomic history of Manipur, the authors concluded that in addition to the availability of more effective contraceptive methods, the changes in attitude "are themselves reflections of social and economic change." Indeed contraceptive uptake was accompanied by a host of factors, including the introduction of modern agricultural technology, institutional innovations (an "uplifting" of the lower castes, improved credit facilities for farmers, and the change to a market economy), as well as the expansion to formal education, particularly among girls. Critical studies of family planning practice like Mamdani's, coupled with subsequent interpretations of change over time, have been rare in the field of anthropology and reproduction (cf. Ward 1986).

Mamdani's (1972:15) comment about lack of this type of analysis was an indictment against the international planning movement at the time: "The almost complete absence of such studies is testimony to the *a priori* assumption of most family planners that birth control programs work."

The swell in gender studies in the 1970s that included international influences helped revitalize feminist scholarship on reproduction. Anthropology's most significant contribution to interpretations of reproduction and, more recently, to population studies, is attributed to the field of medical anthropology and its engagement with political economy. Polgar (1971) was among the first to argue that population growth in underdeveloped countries was tied to Western colonialism and associated pronatalist politics resulting from Western expansion over the last four hundred years. A decade later, Morgan's theoretical and applied work (1989, 1993), based primarily in Costa Rica and influenced by the "world system" approach, shifted the field of medical anthropology into a new mode of analysis, demonstrating how local communities were influenced by national and international forces. This shift gave attention to what Ginsburg and Rapp (1991) dubbed the "politics of reproduction."

Synthesizing the local and the global specifically in Haiti, Farmer (1988b, 1990a, 1990b, 1994, 1999) explained the international influence of power on illness, showing how poverty and other social inequalities alter the patterns and paths of disease distribution and sickness through many complicated mechanisms. Also in Haiti, Brodwin (1996), focusing on moral and medical institutions, portrayed the ways in which indigenous and biomedical health-seeking experiences define peasants' social world, which is also bombarded by global forces in the destitute countryside.

Expanding to the "global" politics of reproduction (Ginsburg and Rapp 1995), the field of fertility and reproduction shifted onto the terrain of power, where policies and politics became central to interpreting fertility. Hartmann (1997) criticized population-control ideology as a way "to avoid addressing deeper causes of underdevelopment, such as inequalities in international relations" (1997:532). Anthropologists provided a grounded perspective by analyzing not only macro-political systems but also micro-social processes through which reproductive health issues were negotiated. Political controversies around the interpretation of maternal mortality (Morsy 1995), contraceptive technologies (Morsy 1993), one-child policies (Anagnost 1995; Greenhalgh and Li, 1995), or the banning of contraceptives and abortions (Kligman 1995) explored women's responses to these policy measures.

Increasingly anthropologists are working to unpack the diverse meanings of gender, power, sexuality, and the politics of reproductive health (Caceres 2000). The recasting of sexuality as socially constructed has thrown a narrow demographic conceptualization into doubt (Lancaster and di Leonardo 1997; Parker, Barbosa, and Aggleton 2000). These studies suggest that transformations in the social and political environments in which sexual and reproductive health decisions are made are central to reproductive rights and service provision. Hirsch's (2003) engaging analysis of gender relations among Mexicans in Atlanta and Mexico situates couples' contraceptive use within the context of sexual and social relationships that change with migratory experiences, over time. Her study shows how the social and cultural meaning of fertility is decidedly more complicated than a demographic preference or health choice. As a study of family planning practice, this case study in Haiti reinforces and builds on these works, linking the social and cultural contexts of fertility to politics—connecting the body and the body politic (Scheper-Hughes and Lock 1987).

A Political Economy of Fertility

Building on inroads made by early family planning critiques and later institutional and feminist critiques of demography and anthropology, Greenhalgh (1988, 1990, 1995) was among the first to apply the political economy framework to the issue of fertility, challenging demography's static interpretations of reproduction. Greenhalgh (1994) proposed a new framework for fertility theory, one rooted in anthropology, that moved demography to a considerably more dynamic plane that incorporates culture, history, gender, and power. The framework accounts for the role of institutions as well as the social actors who live and struggle to survive within them. As social actors, women and men are "active agents of their own reproductive destinies" (Greenhalgh 1994:31). Moving beyond the statistical patterns and frequencies of demography, a political economy of fertility (PEF) teases out the processes that determine population change and looks at how reproduction is determined by larger political, economic, and cultural forces that are constantly in flux. Greenhalgh's original formulation of a PEF was aimed primarily at fertility behaviors. The framework provided a much needed, vital, and dynamic view of how fertility patterns, behavior, and trends could be explained by both micro and macro forces over time.

Recently anthropologists have been engaging more directly with the field of demography. Two edited volumes, *Situating Fertility* (Greenhalgh 1995) and later *Anthropological Demography* (Kertzer and Fricke 1997), present numerous studies that place reproduction within cultural theory and practice. Drawing on new ethnographic and historical research informed by contemporary anthropological theory, Greenhalgh's volume of multidisciplinary works presents a political economy framework threading culture, history, gender, and power into reproductive life. Kertzer and Fricke's volume works more toward a "convergence" of the layered effects of culture, power, and history in both demography and cultural anthropology. However, continued disciplinary tensions over guiding assumptions and methods have left the exploration of integrated approaches to anthropology and demography, like a PEF, largely in the realm of the academy, and disappointingly little effort has been made to apply these findings to current demographic dilemmas.

Studies that have made an effort to apply the political economy approach at the local level to explain the complexity of fertility behaviors have fallen short of encompassing the totality of society's structures: political, economic, and social. Few scholars have critically assessed population program effort that results from misguided population policy. For example, Bledsoe et al. (1994) provide a compelling cultural argument explaining low contraceptive use among rural Gambian women, yet there is little reference to the political or economic forces that may shape individual choice over time. Are traditional birth-spacing practices unaffected by changing national or even global economies? How do Western aid and family planning agencies respond to what is perceived as a persistence of local birth-spacing patterns? And how does this response sit with the recipients of family planning programs?

Where scholars rigorously apply the political economy framework, it is often missing an international perspective, a key level of analysis in view of the fact that that the U.S. government and, more recently, the European Economic Union, are often the predominant funders of reproductive health activities around the world.[13] Renne (1995), for example, links local fertility decision making to national politics in Nigeria. And Weinreb (2001) analyzes how Kenyan politics and culture work to determine differential government spending with "favored" groups receiving a better quality and greater quantity of family planning services. But in both studies questions loom: How do international, structural forces affect national and local levels of discourse and practice? Specifically, what role do development policymakers play in perpetuating fertility decision-making patterns through the often unequal distribution of international aid? How have these issues changed over time?

A more recent work by Renne (2003:208) adds to the literature critiquing underlying assumptions of the demographic transition theory by viewing "how 'people' (population) and 'progress' (local development) are perceived by the residents of a small, rural town in southwestern Nigeria." Demographic constructs come to life in this work—life, death, and numbers take on historical and current significance through everyday practices that Renne respectfully explains through the lens of ritual as well as pragmatism. Interpretations of fertility explain how people confront local and national political and socioeconomic problems. Although this work shows how people both relate and react to ideas about family size, progress (in terms of development), and "actions" of the state, it still falls short of the international global arena even though, as the author states, Nigeria commands significant wealth and therefore power on the continent of Africa. Making the connections between the macro-level political economy and micro-level ethnography would further explain the interconnectedness of structure and agency, so that the full effects of global scale forces might be explained in more corners around the world.

One of the most relevant recent works in anthropology and reproduction is Ali's (2002) study of family planning in Egypt. Squarely acknowledging colonial and postcolonial concerns with populations and demography (here presented as a science of control and governance), Ali views fertility through the perspectives of poor Egyptian citizens. He argues that the family planning program in Egypt seeks to reduce population size while promoting notions of individual choice and self-regulation. Pushing further, he shows how Egypt, as a modernizing state, "uses the family planning program as a pedagogical project to manage its population" (2002:5). Unlike most studies of family planning and reproduction, Ali effectively shows how international recommendations (that accompany development aid)—and internationally spread theories—shape and define population policy in Egypt.

Ali's work in Egypt, like my work in Haiti, considers how globally configured, state-endorsed family planning policy and practices seek, on the one hand, to enhance the range of choices available to women and men but unwittingly, as Ali points out, "create the conditions in which only certain choices can be made" (2002:54). These connections are critical to this study of family planning in Haiti, where the constraints that women and men feel, in the face of deepening poverty fed by political unrest, give new meaning to standard demographic terms such as the "risk" of unwanted fertility. Examining Haiti's population paradox, I use a PEF framework to show how poverty, inequality, gendered discourse, and the politics of family planning hamper not only basic prevention and the provision of reproductive health services but ultimately also people's health and human rights.

Expanding the PEF Framework: Toward Explaining the "Paradox"

To address gaps in some of the previous research and theory, I employ the PEF framework to anchor an ethnographic critique of family planning practice in Cité Soleil. Through attention to local, national, and international activities, a PEF analysis uncovers and explains the social, economic, and political processes that have served to stifle women and men in their quest for reproductive health care. The analysis that unfolds traces the forces of history, gender, power, and culture in creating this supposed paradox. Here, I review these elements individually, though it becomes clear in the ethnographic accounts that follow that they work together in complex ways.

HISTORY. How people construct their reality within historical contexts and the larger political and economic constraints in which they struggle is crucial to a PEF analysis. History, and all of the political nuances that shape it, plays an important role in this analysis because it raises the question of the relationship of fertility and family planning practice to colonialism, neocolonialism, and the powerful international institutions that have resulted from these political arrangements. Underlying this is the basic assumption that "most cultures worldwide are products of a history of appropriations, resistances, and accommodations" (Marcus and Fischer 1986:78). History is used in this work to explain local and global understandings of population movement, growth, and the subsequent family planning interventions designed to contain high fertility. History provides a significant explanation of many of the macro-structural forces that have shaped fertility in Haiti. Trouillot (1990:91), one of Haiti's most prominent political historians, ties these issues together: "The relation between human and natural resources certainly played a catalytic role in the development of what Pierre Charles has called the 'uninterrupted crisis' of Haitian society. The stagnation of the productive forces doomed the system to an eventual breakdown. But demography is not a neutral science: its powers of explanation can only make sense within a socially determined space. Haiti's population growth is handicapped but only within the context of the production and distribution relations imposed by the ruling alliance."

Institutional as well as structural forces have long been at play in shaping Haiti's population and public health sector. Brodwin (1996) effectively documents the lasting effects of American institution building in the realm of public health that began with the American occupation (1915–1934). It was during this period that a highly rationalized health service delivery apparatus was first introduced. The subsequent provision of family planning services blended well with this exogenous system. The implications of these historical trends are significant, and the failure to place Haiti's population problem within this historical context has led to an incomplete analysis and ineffective solutions (see chapter 6).

GENDER. Gender, as an element of the PEF, plays an essential role in understanding fertility, and especially in explaining how reproduction is negotiated in people's lives. The intersection of demography and feminist studies has led to an acknowledgment of gender as a critical element in social, economic, and political settings, including the setting of policy agendas, as at the women's conference in Cairo. These advances have contributed to impressive gains in many countries' efforts to reduce fertility rates and improve women's health over the past several decades. Yet policy failures and shortcomings remain as the HIV epidemic continues, sexually transmitted diseases spread, and numerous subpopulations in most of the world's countries remain untouched or inadequately served by the health systems providing reproductive health services. Additionally, while traditional demographic approaches to the understanding of gender as it relates to sexuality, culture, and power have become part of the endeavor to enhance reproductive health policies and service provision, these analyses too often exclude men as part of the gender system.

In Cité Soleil, the roles of women and men, both individually and in relation to one another, provide the basis for understanding gender and people's relative economic and political power. Issues of economic survival, in the midst of an embargo that all but collapsed Haiti's national economy, provide a useful stage on which to examine forms of discrimination not only against women but equally against men. Like Hirsch (2003) studying sexuality and marriage in transnational Mexican families, the focus in Cité Soleil is on how gender structures people's options and identities. "Gender inequality" says Hirsch (2003:3), "may constrain women's options, but it does not determine them: women and men maneuver within its constraints, as they do within those of race and class." In Cité Soleil, gender crosses into the household, the family planning center, and the community where popular political organizing focuses on what residents viewed as inappropriate reproductive health care.

POWER. An institutional analysis of family planning, with power at its center, brings to the fore critical issues as they relate to bodies and the body politic. Power appears in different guises throughout this work. "In any society, there are manifold relations of power which permeate, characterize and constitute the social body" (Foucault 1980:93). Foucault's characterization of power is deeply relevant as it weaves its way through the multiple levels of the political economy analysis. As women and men negotiate their positions with each other and within a society that strips them both of their reproductive as well as human rights, it becomes clear that "individuals are always in the position of simultaneously undergoing and exercising this power" (Foucault 1980:98).

Various medical anthropologists have described the workings of power in reproductive health (Farmer 2003; Gupta 2002; Molyneux 1985, Parker et al. 2000). But one of "the problem[s] with power in anthropological studies," begins Ellen (2002:250), "is that it comes and goes depending on the subject under investigation, the level and unit of analysis selected, and the methodology employed." In this study, power is a consistent and central element. Local power relations in the community between women and men, clients and their providers, and community organizers and antidemocratic forces are central to explaining why family planning as a seemingly benign public health intervention failed. These locally generated meanings provide an understanding of how power and reproduction interact as political and economic mechanisms of control at the level of the individual, community, nation state, region, and increasingly the globe.

In Haiti, demographers and development experts' steady preoccupation with implementing family planning programs, hitting contraceptive quotas, and reaching "desired fertility levels" has ensured that they have overlooked local resistance to using family planning, itself nested in many forms of power. For residents in Cité Soleil, nearly every primary health care intervention offered by the local nongovernmental organization came to embody a form of domination. Residents' resistance and revolt exposes how the absence of power—or disempowerment—has helped fuel unwanted fertility in this community. At the national level, caught in a devolving political economy, Haitians find themselves increasingly dependent on international aid but with no control over the terms and definitions of this assistance. Power then becomes both a dimension and an explanatory factor of why and how forty years of international efforts to bring family planning to this impoverished nation have failed to thrive.

CULTURE. In Haiti, a notable trend in evaluation reports, survey writeups, and general assessments of fertility and family planning programs written by experts is to cite "culture" as a largely undefined and problematic notion that keeps fertility high. Program failure is defined in terms of cultural barriers, cultural attitudes, cultural preferences, cultural practices, and cultural traditions—all noted as obstacles. Culture frequently becomes a way to explain inaction, since culture is perceived as slow to change. Most demographic theory, policy, or evaluation does little to explain cultural change or processes. Greenhalgh (1990, 1994) suggests that to "untangle" cultural processes is key. Explaining the causal, culturally embedded mechanisms underlying fertility choices and behavior is central to this study of family-planning practice and policy.

Employing history, gender, power, and culture, a PEF looks at how reproduction—extended here to include family planning and its core practices in the field—is determined by these larger forces constantly in flux. The chapters that follow wind in and out of the homes, the clinic, and the Cité Soleil community, shedding light on previously misunderstood reproductive strategies. At the local level, the PEF shows how efforts to engage women as liberated contraceptive "users" are entirely misconceived, unveiling the ways that "gender empowerment"—as it is often employed in family planning circles—has little to do with people's realities. Inside the clinic, the medicalization of clinic encounters and fundamentally serious issues around what development experts promote as the "quality of care," make this center an unlikely place for women to find the health care they need. At the community level, PEF analysis forcefully shows how social, economic, and even political structures dominate and determine the parameters of survival, especially as they relate to reproduction. At the national and regional levels, demography's diagnosis for aggressive family planning activities is revealed as highly inappropriate, given Haiti's past and present history. The analysis shows how the provision of family planning, too often viewed as a simple and pragmatic biomedical intervention, is both complex and undeniably political. Placing fertility and family planning practice in Haiti within this broad, multilevel, process-oriented framework helps explain the population "paradox" that has stymied observers for so long.

3

Gender and Survival

Living on the Edge in Cité Soleil

Oh we are in deep. When a man gives you a child now, he leaves, without ever looking back. It's a huge injustice. You wish that he had killed you instead. And when you're pregnant, I don't need to tell you about the hunger, bare feet on the ground, everything in your body cries out. You need to pay for your house and, if you can't, they throw you out. Pay for the house, pay for everything. There have been times when I would just stop and ask God, "Why did you make me?"

–Marie Ange, Cité Soleil resident, 1994

I can honestly tell you–with no jobs, no food and, in the end, no love–life today is worse than death itself. I think I'll get more respect when I am dead.

–Harold, Cité Soleil resident, 2003

In Cité Soleil, the household domain is highly private and seldom understood by outsiders wishing to improve the conditions of this community. The division of resources and responsibilities between men and women is largely determined when households are first set up, and it is here that strategies for survival are conceived and coordinated. It is inside households that power, authority, and conflict define the contours of gender relations. Households are terrains of bargaining, and bargaining in turn works through cultural rules. The contracts that result play a part in complex gender processes.

My years of building rapport and friendships made forays into Cité Soleil homes a natural part of this research. What I subsequently discovered adds to a very small body of information about urban survival strategies in Haiti. Households are central to this analysis for another important reason: because the household is where nearly all subjects of the study insisted we talk. Residents were at once proud of their humble homes and shamed by the fact that they could not offer me a cola or even a chair to sit on. Once the always polite formalities

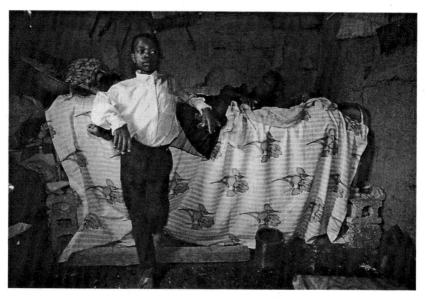

One-room home, Cité Carton, a section of Cité Soleil

were finished, we would sit on cement blocks hauled in from outside, or sit together, legs dangling on the edge of a bed made lumpy by its corn-husk stuffing. It was only in the privacy of these homes that the most hidden of human agendas appeared.

Concepts of unions and households, as defined by demographers in surveys, paint a broad picture with neatly defined clean categories delineating who heads a household in Haiti. In reality, standard household definitions are far from the norm, and they are rarely stable. Unions in Haiti are often shifting, and these shifts often occur, as this chapter shows, around pecuniary issues (cf. Guyer 1988). There are, in reality, many forces—social, economic, and political—that bombard poor Haitian households these days, as well as in other parts of the world. Setel (1999), working in Tanzania, shows how traditional ideas and practices related to sexuality and fertility are changing in the face of modernity, biomedicine, and HIV/AIDS. There are similar changes under way in Haiti, and these are made all the more glaring by the effects of structural and state-sponsored violence against the poor.

The Making of Haitian Homes: Tradition and Honor

Anyone entering one of the cramped homes in Cité Soleil feels what residents call *lamizè* (misery). Nearly every roof is made of tin, which traps the heat from the relentless rays of the sun and makes homes feel like ovens. As a courtesy, I was frequently provided a neatly folded towel or rag to wipe the sweat from my brow as it accumulated within minutes of entering. Residences in this sample were one story high and typically had one or two rooms, the most spacious measuring forty square meters (approximately 430 sq feet). Just over half the respondents (51 percent) lived in two rooms, while the others (49 percent) lived in a single room. Inside these cramped and stifling quarters an average of eight people ate and slept daily. Many of the houses doubled as businesses: One was a dressmaker's shop during the day, and another served as a kitchen (called a "popular restaurant") during the day and a brothel at night.

Houses are made of rudimentary materials, many of which are recycled. Typical structures are made of cement blocks (74 percent), wooden planks (17 percent), tin or straw (9 percent each). Floors are made of cement (91 percent) or earth (9 percent). Doors are usually made of tin or wood, and barbed wire often defines the front entrance, fashioned like a gate, in an effort to keep vandals at bay. Houses are generally dark and dank inside, for lack of electricity. Crude windows have shutters, but they are usually sealed to keep roving spirits away. One of the community's poorest sites is Cité Carton (Cardboard City), a neighborhood where during the rainy season life is especially grueling. After a rainfall, residents search for days for dry cardboard and, if and when they are successful, fasten the material to long wooden poles that serve as the house's structure.

Inside most houses there is one bed, raised on at least four cinder blocks to keep it dry. A double bed typically sleeps a minimum of four people and sometimes up to six children and two adults. Clothing, if there are spare pieces, is often hung from a rope attached to rafters above the bed to create a curtain and a sense of privacy when sleeping. Sleeping is rarely a rejuvenating event, since living quarters are so confined. Fritznel, a forty two-year-old male, spent a good deal of time describing how twelve people (all but two are adults or young adults) managed to sleep in his one-room home. He began by telling me how difficult it was to breathe at night, and then he carefully described the following configuration: three slept on the platform loft he built (*men li cho anpil*—but it is very hot [up there]), four on a double bed, one on a cot and three on a mat on the floor. He ended his description with a pause, and then said, "Sleeping in Haiti is dangerous." Where space is even more limited, residents of Cité Soleil opt for one of several possibilities: sleeping in shifts (whereby people take four- to six-hour sleeping shifts and walk around the community when awake) or eking out space on tables, inside oil barrels, or on straw or cardboard mats placed on any remaining dry surface. Rat bites are common in these conditions.

Poverty, however, does not keep residents from decorating their property. Everything in the Haitian household is carefully and strategically placed. Favored decorations are plastic flowers (blue roses are popular) and cheap imported vases from China. Tables are typically dressed with brightly colored vinyl coverings.

Shelves may have perfume bottle boxes or small, empty plastic shampoo bottles also used as decoration. An occasional ashtray from the Bahamas or even a fragment of a bygone mirror can be found neatly displayed. Old dusty televisions, rarely functional, are often crammed into corners, and almost every house has a transistor radio, often playing when there is electricity. Photos of Jesus and outdated calendars are sealed in plastic bags to protect them from the dirt, and hung on the walls. In several houses I noticed wardrobe suitcases hanging from the wall, as if in anticipation of traveling. Wallpaper is often ingeniously created from pages of *El Nacional, Sports Illustrated, Paris Match*, or American clothing catalogues.

Other typical home furnishings include one cabinet and one or two chairs (usually made of metal and crafted in Haiti). Inside the cabinet, or stored in a corner of the house, are kitchen utensils such as two cooking pots, a *recho* (three-legged metal brazier used to hold burning charcoal and a cooking pot), three or four cooking spoons, a few plastic bowls and metal cups, spoons that serve as eating utensils, and one or two large plastic basins for dishwashing and laundry. Water, when available, is typically stored in large plastic buckets in the corners of houses. Linens consist of one set of sheets, one or two face cloths, and one large towel that is used communally.

Courtship and Union: Love in the Haitian Household

The foundation upon which the traditional Haitian household is built is the "union"—a term demographers use to describe how couples pair for reproductive purposes. Several sociologists and anthropologists have sought to define the multiple types of relationships, or unions, which unite Haitian women and men (see Allman 1980; Lowenthal 1984, 1987; Neptune-Anglade 1986), though most of these works are based on conditions in rural Haiti. Because Haiti remains the most rural of all Latin American countries, it is not surprising that the majority of literature on sexuality or gender is based in the rural milieu. The majority of respondents in this study were born in the countryside and migrated to the city hoping to improve their economic status; for women as well as men, this implied finding a partner, setting up a home, and having a child. The degree to which these relationships change in urban Haiti is notable.

Allman's classification of different types of union is useful to situate the reader in the complex arena of Haitian union status. The author states that *renmen* (to like/love, 6 percent) *fiyanse* (to be engaged, 6 percent) and *viv avèk* (to live with, though on a sporadic basis, 20 percent) generally do not involve cohabitation and only minimal economic support. Other major types of unions, *mariye* (marriage, 17 percent) and *plase* (common-law, 34 percent) are the strongest of unions and normally involve cohabitation and economic support. *Divòse/vèf* (divorced/widowed, 17 percent) were also reported by women in Cité Soleil. Any one of these unions can produce a child, though children are more commonly the result of marriage or common-law unions.

Talking about sex and sexuality is widely accepted in most parts of Haiti. Haitians view sex as a natural, normal, and necessary part of life. Expressions of sexuality begin at a very young age. When asked about their very first sexual contact, men and women told me about *jwèt timoun*—a widely practiced game of sexual initiation that begins around five or six years and lasts until about eight or nine years, when children "imitate" their parents, and boys "make love" to girls. This is, of course, all in jest. Respondents confirmed that penetration occurs but pregnancy does not, because neither boy nor girl is *fòme*—or mature. Social and economic pressure to mate after puberty, however, is high, as evidenced by rates of fertility among young girls and women: by seventeen years, 19 percent of all women have already had a baby or are pregnant. The proportion increases to 31 percent by the time Haitian girls are nineteen years old (EMMUS III 2000). The Haitian proverb *mariyaj 20, pitit 21*—marriage at 20, children at 21—remains culturally and statistically germane today.

As in many places around the world, a significant part of male identity in Haiti is bound up in sexuality, both in terms of men's public bravado and their ability to follow through, find a suitable partner, and ultimately maintain the relationship. Before setting up a household, Haitian men and women enter into a period of formal courtship that is based on a time-honored and traditional process of establishing relationships. "You sweat and you sweat and you sweat, until you succeed," explains Jean Robert referring to the rules of Haitian courtship. For men, winning the favor of a Haitian woman is, like most strategies in Haitian society, a well-calculated one. It requires great patience and leaves decision making, at least superficially, to women. Most men in this study unabashedly contend that they always win, because no challenge is too great when it comes to love.

As if to affirm their sexuality and their expressed sexual needs, nearly every man interviewed would state early on in the conversation, *gason pa ka rete san fi* (a man can't be without a woman). When the topic of courtship and sex came up, so did the laughs and smiles. Men enjoy talking about sex; it provides them with a strong sense of who they are in an otherwise marginalized and demeaning world. When asked about homosexuality, all men in the sample acknowledged that it existed but also indicated that it was aberrant behavior, as one man said: *pami diri gen woch* (in the rice grains you'll always find a pebble). Pressure to perform as a man within the heterosexual relationship is strong; from a young age men are expected to fulfill their roles as *filè-s* (flirts). Schwartz (2000:117), working in rural Haiti, corroborates my findings in Cité Soleil: "Men who do not express overt interest in sex by propositioning young women are thought of as handicapped or deficit, they are teased by people of both sexes and all ages, even children, and taunted with names like *djèjè* (imbecile) and *masisi* (homosexual), the latter being considered an abomination that qualifies a person [in rural areas] among the ranks of the insane."

For women, "You just need to buy them things—sandals, a dress, sodas, chocolates, and flowers—it's easy to win them over." As the Haitian saying goes, *pou gen fi, fo gen lajan* (in order to have a woman, you must have money) or the more derogatory *fi konn manje gason* (women eat men up), meaning they take all their money. In almost all cases, material circumstances dictate. René Mark, a man who inherited the title of pastor (he was an assistant to a pastor when the pastor died), considers himself quite religious and very respectful of women. And yet, when he referred to women, he equated them first to furniture, "You want your woman like a good piece of furniture, beautiful and long lasting," and then later to cars: "If you want a nice car, then you need to invest." And so begins the process of forming unions in Haiti.

Women were less effusive about their sexuality, though it is also central to their identity. While being *sèksi* (sexy) is important for many Haitian women, it was not described (or recalled) in nearly as playful or joyous terms. Often, older women will initiate younger men into their first sexual experience, indicating some degree of sexual power that women hold over men. And women can be quite aggressive about finding the right man. Several women told me about different ways to snare eligible men "apart from looking pretty in church" or "buying a magic spell" from the local *vodou* healer. One woman described in great detail her most effective love potion: a meal of rice and beans, using water in which she had washed her underwear in as the basis of her recipe. This can either win a man over, or poison him in cases where the man is not receptive to her love. If poisoning occurs, the only known antidote, according to men, is for the man's mother to make a similar meal, or to make fruit juice, this time using the mother's underwear-washing water to make the juice.

The power and centrality of women's sexuality is illustrated blatantly in songs and dances of Haiti. In the countryside, where dance troupes called *teyat* are still common, Schwartz (2000) found that young girls ages 12 to 20 practice daily dancing and singing, with the themes revolving primarily around sexuality.

A place, I need a place
To spin myself around [get wild]
Underneath my house [underneath my dress]
I have an adult [my genitals are mature]
Who is shaking me [making me so I can hardly stand myself]

Look here, it is mango season
Look here, the mangos are sweet and beautiful
Good day, young lady, I say to you good day
It is a plantain that has come to make things sweet
    —(Schwartz [his translation] 2000:115)

In Cité Soleil, the rough contours of urban survival have nearly disintegrated the prevalence of spontaneous dancing troupes like those Schwartz described in rural Haiti. Young girls and boys have little time for leisure, and contribute to the household from an early age. Provocative dancing and lyrics are, however, still a significant part of urban life, but they are generally expressed during celebrations such as Mardi Gras and Rara, Haiti's pre-Lenten celebrations. McAllister (2002) devotes an entire chapter to the "irreverent vulgarity" that spills forth during these important pre-Lenten and Lenten ceremonies. References to fertility abound, immodesty reigns, and men, women, and children have a great deal of fun with *betiz* (a form of Haitian Creole speech full of sexual innuendos and used during Rara songs): "Take out the dick, stick the dick under the clitoris," "When I see you I want to come. The heat of your pussy makes me not able to come," or the absurdity of "Go roll titties. Go roll your mama's titties." These lyrics almost always deal with women, sexuality, and money.

Women's power in the realm of sexuality is almost always directed toward financial gain. Every woman interviewed told me they were not in a relationship for love or sexual enjoyment. Rather, unions help women survive. Single women have every right to use their sexuality to acquire material support from their paramours and, as we will see, having children is women's major source of bargaining power in relationships. Women are conscious of the value of their genitalia, as reflected in these references: *byen pa m* (my goods/assets), *peyi m* (my country), and *tè m* (my land), to name a few. And genitalia are used to negotiate with men, throughout the relationship, though not always successfully or to a woman's advantage.

It is common and generally accepted for men to have several partners at one time and to have children with several women. Some scholars of Haiti argue that sex ratios are low, meaning that there are more women than men in Haiti, and this could be interpreted as a reason for polygamy, but my research indicates that gendered cultural reasons have more to bear on this phenomenon. Schwartz (2000:260) goes on to explain that polygamy, in rural Haiti, "while not legal . . . [is] different from the "extramarital affair" in that 1) it is public, 2) efforts are made to produce children in all the unions, 3) the man continues to perform his role as provider, planting gardens and tending livestock for all of the women, and 4) the women are expected to remain sexually faithful to the man." Acknowledging these preordained rights, men were very comfortable discussing their sexual histories, including the number of former and current partners. All of the men interviewed had at least two current partners (and often more), except for one older man who was going blind. Woldy, a handsome Twenty-nine-year-old, had three children, each with different women, and three casual partners on the side. He explained it like this: "Men have their needs; it entertains me." Thirty-two-year-old Maxo had three partners: his *madanm mariye* (married wife), a *ti renmen* (a "little love") and a woman *andeyò* (in the countryside).

Women are traditionally not afforded the same sexual freedom as men, and most of the women interviewed expressed this as a violation of their rights. They would look at me, when I asked why Haitian society allowed this, and they would inevitably begin their analysis with a shake of the head and say, "*se pa jis*" (it's not fair). However, if a woman is not in union and not supported by another man, then generally she is allowed to engage in an affair with a man who offers financial rewards for her keep. Women rely primarily on serial monogamy (Auguste 1995), with established unions often disintegrating after the birth of the child (when men are unable to follow through with financial obligations). As a result, most women in Cité Soleil have a different father for each child.

Gendered Contracts and Expectations

Although there are aberrations from the norm, residence in urban Haiti is generally neolocal, meaning that new couples establish new households when they make a commitment to one another. Inevitably, over time, this evolves into a matrilocal system where the women stay put, essentially because they are responsible for their children, and the men move on. Where shared households are the norm, there is a strict division between women's work and men's work, and these gendered divisions are tied up in the expected gender roles that Haitian society dictates.

Women's work (*travay fanm*) is primarily domestic: washing, ironing, preparing food, sweeping, caring for children, and maintaining the household. Men demand these domestic duties and childbearing from women, and many are appreciative. Felix, a school teacher dressed in rags, is unabashed by his dependence on his wife: "Women are men's saviors. I can't hide it," he says, looking me straight in the eyes. "If she were not around, I wouldn't eat." Men's work (*travay gason*) is often more "fix-it" oriented: cutting bushes (if there are any), performing yard work (often shared with women), replacing and fixing lights (when they have them), and repairing broken pieces of furniture and general carpentry jobs. All of this work and other expectations are part of an understood, though rarely openly discussed, contract that women and men enter into when a union begins.

A great deal of this unspoken household contract is imbued with expectations. When asked what men expect of women, Pierre, who has fathered six children (four in the countryside and two in the city), said, "lots of things." Sitting on a wooden chair that is missing half of its woven seat, he leaned back. Crammed into sandals at least two sizes too small for his calloused feet, he laughed confidently, "love, cooking, washing, and ironing." Then, after a short pause he said, "and of course having a child." His response was nearly identical to all the other men interviewed in this study.

Remarkably, all of the men interviewed in this study neglected to mention that women are also generally required to bring in some income to the household.

The omission of women's very small, but significant, earning power may reflect an unconscious denial of the fact that without women's earned income, most Haitian households would not survive.

The Wealth of the Poor

Since women look to men primarily, and often exclusively, for economic support, a man who woos a woman is generally successful if he can offer help for the children she already has. Three women said that sexual caresses were important to them, though a man's ability to bring in income to help maintain a household was an overriding priority. During times of escalated violence, many women indicated that a man afforded them some increased security, though one woman commented, "but we are all poor, and these days, man or woman, danger is everywhere." Overall, women in Cité Soleil had very basic eligibility requirements for potential partners: good health and the ability to work. A good partner is based on the idealized concept of a *nèg seriyè* (a solid man): a man who brings in an income and provides for his partner and their children. Women hope that he will not run around with or make promises to other women. If he does, he is a *vakabon* (a good-for-nothing, shameless scoundrel), and if a woman makes it unpleasant enough for him, he can be evicted (or will leave on his own accord, often to his mother's home or another girlfriend's place). This is the ideal, but increasingly, in the face of reduced earning power, women are less likely to evict men in hopes that they might garner some economic support.

Bound up in these gendered roles are the ideals of motherhood and fatherhood, where both parents contribute to the provision of the very basic needs of children: food, clothing, and shelter. Eschewing these roles is unheard of, since childlessness, according to Lowenthal (1987:309), "is a virtually untenable status, ultimately undermining efforts to live a proper and meaningful life." These are standards that men and women still attempt to conform to, even in the face of a dramatically changed reality marked by a devastating decline in earning capacity. After all, as the widely used Haitian proverb goes, *ti moun se richès pòv malèrè* (children are the wealth of the poor). Or as Jude, an old toothless resident of Cité Soleil who has been unemployed for years, said to me: "*Yon moun pa gen moso pitit pa moun*" (a person who doesn't have a child is not a person).

In all unions, producing children marks a critical entry into adulthood (see Lowenthal 1984).[1] And children serve a clear purpose, even in urban areas. Women and men in this study are quick to rattle off the "work" that children, as young as five years of age, are expected to do, including carrying water, running errands, helping sell in the markets, washing dishes, making meals, washing clothes, ironing, and so on. Life in urban Haiti depends heavily on a fragile hand-to-mouth existence, and children play vitally important roles in the process of barely sustaining households on the economic margins.

While all parents fight to see their children survive, the odds are stacked against Haitian babies from the start. Infant mortality rates for under one year of age and up to five years of age are the highest in this hemisphere (EMMUS III 2000). Having more than one child helps guarantee a family's overall survival rate. This is reflected in the proverb I often heard: *Si gen jè pete, gen lòt* (if you lose one eye, you have another).

Apart from working around the home, children as young as seven and eight years old are charged with watching younger children to free adults and older siblings to work outside of the home, improving the chances that another income source will prove fruitful. Gender roles are defined even at this early point in life. Girls typically help with the travay fanm that they will be expected to perform for men later in life. Interestingly, boys also learn many of the same skills that young girls learn, but when they enter adolescence, they are no longer expected to perform these duties. All children learn some form of marketing skills and usually help their mothers on market days. Either way, making ends meet is critical, and children help. During the fieldwork period, garbage foraging was a common job for family members as young as eight years old. Mothers would tie small aprons with big pockets to the waists of children who climbed on heaps of garbage in search of leftover food and recyclables. In 1994, when the U.S. forces returned then President Aristide to Haiti, this work became increasingly competitive since, as one child indicated, *"blan yo bay bèl fatra"* (foreigners provide beautiful garbage).

In addition to what they contribute in labor, children remain potential investments. Although their prospects for attaining even basic education are not very strong, parents hold out hope that at least one child will make it in Haiti—or get to Miami.[2] In conversations with parents—both women and men—it was striking how much hope remained vested in children in spite of the devastating economic outlook. Men interviewed always had high aspirations for their children, as if oblivious to the financial and class obstacles that Haitians know all too well. When asked what they expected from their children, apart from household duties, they would project into the future: "If God is willing," it would always begin, "my child could be a doctor, a lawyer, or an engineer." Indeed, children remain Haitians' only form of social security. And, in many cases, children are the only thing that poor Haitians can claim as their own, since they are denied virtually every other right to ownership as citizens. And of course, wrapped up in myriad large and looming political, economic, and cultural forces, there are also very human emotional forces at work: Children are cherished and loved.

Understanding these traditional and honored expectations is fundamental to explaining, later in this chapter, how economic and political forces are eroding the foundation of Haitian households. Clearly, the ideal roles for men and women are nearly impossible to fulfill. Living up to cultural ideals of "responsible" relationships has become virtually impossible in the midst of Haiti's crippling political economy. Lived experiences and contested identities emerge in distinctly gendered ways for men and women and are critical to understanding reproductive behavior, the implications of which are deeply relevant to family-planning policy and programs.

"The Meaning of Macho": Being a Man in Port-au-Prince

Critical of the academic, anthropological fascination with the "macho" concept, Matthew Gutmann's (1996) work in Mexico deconstructs the notion of a unitary man, an urban man, or even an urban working-class man, and shows that even etymologically the terms "macho" and "machismo" have meanings that change over time, class, and space. Interviews with men during a period of great political instability and economic uncertainty show how machismo in the Haitian context is constantly changing amid the persisting patterns of gender inequality. Gender in Cité Soleil is constrained by inequality and stereotypes and is marked by change and contradiction.

Men and Work

Apart from talking in detail about their sexual lives, in conversation men deliberated a great deal about employment. Earning power is key to men's identity, since it is what makes them desirable and useful to a household on the edge of survival. Men take their prescribed role of breadwinner seriously and would often reiterate in various ways, *kom gason se mwen menm ki chèf kay la* (as a man, it's me who is the head of the house). In many places in the world men have considerably more control over economic resources than do women, thus giving them an upper hand on all household decisions. To be sure, in Cité Soleil, when men find jobs in construction, for example, they can earn from ten to a hundred times more than a market woman selling mangoes (de Zalduondo et al. 1995). For this reason, most men spend much of their time searching for work. Day workers leave home around 5:00 a.m. to seek work and often return by 10:00 a.m. if unsuccessful. Construction workers with tools or laborers carrying shovels walk from job to job and from dawn to dusk in search of work (Fass 1980). In the mid-1990s, however, unemployment hovered around 70 percent. During this period and continuing through the present day, the process of searching for a job in urban Haiti is not an easy task.[3]

When men find jobs, they always take on an increased risk of morbidity and mortality. A physician working in Cité Soleil told me that at any given time, 80 percent of all men present with hernias, directly associated with the heavy loads that men carry and pull. Observers of Haiti are usually stunned to see what a single human being can pull. A man hauling a *bourèt* (a large wheelbarrow-type cart), rents the bourèt for about 50 cents a day and is paid for the number and weight of the sacks that he pulls; he needs to pull several loads a day to make even a tiny profit of $1. If the loads are heavy, he has to pay another man to push in the back.

The Cité Soleil wharf—an area where a long dock serves as a port for trade—is another source for jobs, though few are high-paying, and all are taxing. Men carry huge bags of prepared charcoal off the boats and store it in Cité Charbon (Charcoal City), a community just adjacent to the wharf area. This neighborhood stores charcoal not immediately snatched up by vendors. Everything there—the earth, the homes, and many of the people—are thickly coated in black charcoal dust. Several hours of this backbreaking work will yield under US$1. Others, who are fishermen by trade, sew nets during the day, and at night, around 6 p.m., they rent motors and sails and take to the seas, returning home at 10 a.m. so that their partners can hawk fish to residents. This is dangerous work and requires that fishermen go farther and farther out to find fish, since Haiti's seas are over-fished and coral reefs are dying from the runoff of the now denuded mountains that make up most of Haiti's territory. All of these jobs are considered low-class—hard manual labor for the uneducated.

Men in the study who were apprenticed in a trade or had some education were employed at one point in their lives, but no one had steady paid work. For example, at one point in 2002, I interviewed a mechanic, two indigenous healers, a schoolteacher, a tap tap driver, a "pastor," and two health-care workers. All of these men were very proud of their stated occupations and spoke at

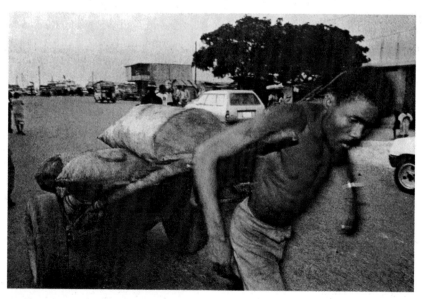

Hauling charcoal, Cité Soleil

length about how they acquired their skills. But in each case, when I probed to ask about actual earning power, shame shrouded their eyes. The healer told me that no one could pay for herbal concoctions any more and that his business was suffering. The schoolteacher told me that he was last paid six months ago and that his salary, which has not increased since 1992, was US$31 every three months. He has taught on credit, since no one can afford tuition. He added, looking away from me, as if the facts were too much to bear, "The children are too hungry to learn anyhow." The tap tap driver had also worked only sporadically, because gasoline prices had increased so dramatically and transportation strikes had made work impossible.[4] The pastor told me that although his church held services, people were too poor to give offerings. And one of the health-care workers, on the government payroll, had not been paid for over six months.

Men as Providers

For men, gender relations are straightforward: As earning power drops, so too does their ability to fulfill their conjugal contract. Living up to these economic ideals has never been easy for the Haitian man. The extent to which some men try to be responsible is impressive and wrapped up in the region's economy. As if to differentiate himself from the common image of Haitian men as good-for-nothings, Woldy, the young man who had three children by three different women, started his tale like this: "I am different; I want to help all of my women." When his job as a tap tap driver failed to pan out, he contacted his sister, Martine, who lives illegally in Guadaloupe. At that point, Woldy pulled out her picture from an otherwise empty wallet to show me. "Her beauty," he claims, gesturing to her pretty face, "landed her a position in a jewelry store." This meant that she could send about US$200 every three months, to Woldy's landless parents in Haiti. The parents then divide the cash among Woldy and two other brothers. Another brother in New York (also undocumented, but using false papers) had collected disability from a car accident and he, too, was contributing to the family fund. Anxious to find work to help support his three children and their mothers, Woldy invested US$300 for a one-way ticket to Guadaloupe, where he hoped his sister could help him find a job. But Woldy had no such luck. "I felt like an imprisoned animal," he recounted. "Cooped up in a house all day because it was a period when immigration was cracking down." After two months of waiting and hoping, Woldy returned to Haiti for US$250 on a second one-way ticket. When the brother in New York was subsequently deported and his sister broke up with her partner, Woldy and his family hit an economic crisis. Martine's most recent news, that she was dating a French man, was a promising possibility—one that the entire family was focusing on. Shaking his head and looking away from me, Woldy's anxiety over his poverty was tangible.

In conversation, all the men were deeply troubled by their inability to fulfill their conjugal contracts. They would drop their heads, look at the ground, and hold their heavy brows in their hands when the subject of their poverty came up. Even so, most held on tight to their male identity. Witness Julmis, a thirty-two-year-old *houngan* (vodou priest), who has a very strong sense of himself as healer and provider both to his community and to his two partners. Houngans never fear for their lives, he explained, because they serve a critical role to everyone. When describing his profession, he too pulled out his symbolically thin wallet and showed me a card that honored him as a member of the National African Religious Conference. His clients, he told me, would often come to resolve social problems, and he focuses frequently on reconciliation between men and women. He makes charms and gives advice, all of which he learned from his father and in his dreams. For most visits he charges about 250 gourdes, or about US$5.50.

At the time of our interview Julmis was married with six children living in Cité Soleil in two different households. He also admitted to having two other women in different parts of Port-au-Prince whom he visited from time to time. In exchange for sexual favors he paid these casual partners small amounts of cash, but even this was difficult. He had some clients but very sporadically; his *peristil* (a temple) in Soley 17, one of Cité Soleil's politically charged neighborhoods, looked worn and spirit-free. This observation was confirmed when he told me he had not performed a ceremony in over seven months. When I asked how a man making so little income could provide for six children—with a couple of women on the side—his bravado diminished and he described a "panic" that runs around the body. "This is why everything is so crazy now," he continued. He looked at me with suddenly angry, piercing eyes and said, "Look, if you want to live these days, you've got to be bad." When I asked what "bad" meant, he referred to others he knows, members of gangs who kill for money or booze in drug deals, "the ones paid by the people in power."

Still, Julmis insisted that in spite of these troubling times, the ability to fulfill the Haitian male role was not deteriorating. During the course of our conversation, however, he eventually moved from a place of pride to a place of sheer humility: "I'll tell you how bad it is. There are times now when I can't even go home to my wife. How can I go home, after a day of loitering, and ask for a meal in front of my children, when I know that they haven't eaten all day? They are lucky some days if they have a single piece of bread and sugar water. What am I left to do? Instead I'll go to someone else's home, or I'll visit the mother of my other children, or one of my girlfriends, and they'll provide food for me when I need it. I'll tell you, things are not easy. *Chagren touye nou* (the grief is killing us)."

Men and Sex

Consistently, men referred to needing to keep busy during the day with "distractions." When I asked what men did to distract themselves, they listed several typical male activities such as betting at the lottery or playing dominoes, a favorite game in Haiti. But many of them noted that under changing economic conditions, they were performing household duties (*travay fanm*) more regularly. Several men indicated that they would help around the house ironing or washing dishes or play with the children while women were out marketing. *Lavi a chanje* (life is changing), they would say, indicating that men had to help, since market women were the only ones who could make money.

All the men (except for one devout Christian) also noted that alcohol and sexual relations (outside of their main partners) were two important additional forms of distraction. These declarations of sex as an important distraction always followed after I pressed men about performing travay fanm. It was almost as if men could not tolerate my questions that so clearly deconstructed their version of traditional male roles. Men clearly said that maintaining their identity as men meant taking risks that are known to be hazardous to their health (Doyal 2000). Alcohol-related accidents and sexually transmitted diseases, according to men, are on the rise. "What else can we do?" asked Friznel, shrugging his shoulder in defeat and drunk at 10 a.m. on *kleren* (sugarcane alcohol) when I visited him in his extremely modest dwelling. Haitian men argued in no uncertain terms that drinking alcohol and other high-risk behaviors are direct products of society, a socially created problem in response to the undignified meaning of "macho" in Cité Soleil.

Within a political economy framework, it becomes clear that the structural forces within Haitian society have literally stripped men of their most basic asset: that of being a responsible partner and provider. In an effort to hold onto what little sense of masculinity they may have, sexuality plays an increasingly important role. Not only do men have fewer resources in a continually dismal economy but, because of multiple unions, they also split an already thin supply of cash across several households. This means that short-term liaisons with extraconjugal partners are considerably easier to obtain, since they require only small financial investments (de Zalduondo et al. 1995).[5] Though extraconjugal sexual relationships may be financially more feasible, longer-term relationships are still coveted because of the domestic benefits they afford.

In 2003, when I returned to Haiti to interview a second group of men, things had grown worse. During interviews men made it clear that their lives were under siege. Constant political instability and economic deterioration have led to a general disintegration, leaving men with even fewer employment options than before. When I asked about work, almost all the men claimed that there was really only one type of lucrative job left in Cité Soleil—"work for the state," a not-so-coded way of referring to the gang members, with specific political affiliations to those in power. The buying and selling of drugs has consumed the community. These troubling political and economic times have worn the social fabric of Cité Soleil down to its barest threads.

Several younger men told me that they were postponing a formal union because they couldn't afford to buy the chocolates or flowers to woo their girl-friends. Jean Robert, who has fathered five children and has one casual sexual partner in addition to his main partner, reframes the economic problem in a profoundly social way. He said, "*nou pa gen renmen ankò* (we don't have love any more). Everything is an exchange. You pay them for sex and they pay you for sex. Men go for women, women go for men, women for women and men for men. It doesn't matter any more; you take what you can get. What does this mean? A man can't be a man. We've been reduced to animals."

Love and Loss: Being a Woman in Port-au-Prince

While Haitian men, as partners and sons, clearly suffer from the effects of pervasive poverty, the unfortunate truth is that poverty in Haiti is gendered. Indicators of female disadvantage are etched into the country's legal system. The Haitian constitution, for instance, requires that a woman turn over all that she inherits to her husband. Women in business are, according to the law, required to receive authorization from their husbands to run the business, and husbands are responsible for helping repay debt, though this rarely happens in practice. In reality this law is not applied, and the burden of debt repayment is often shouldered by poor women. The majority of poor women in all types of unions, and their children born from these unions, remain unrecognized by the Haitian judicial system. Marriage is the only legal union recognized in Haiti. The legal code punishes women more severely than men if they are caught committing adultery; the age for sexual consent is eighteen years for boys, but fifteen years for girls (François 1995; Pierre-Pierre 1995).

Other indicators of women's disadvantage are captured in large-scale health and demographic surveys. In 1990, the Population Crisis Committee rated the condition of women in the Western Hemisphere, placing Haiti at the very bottom of the scale, lagging behind Guatemala, Bolivia, Honduras, and Nicaragua (IDB 1990). A decade later things have not significantly improved. Documenting worldwide conditions for mothers, Haiti ranked 96th of 117 countries (Save the Children 2003). Results show that both Haitian girls and women have higher rates of mortality, poorer nutritional status, and lower rates of literacy and education than their male counterparts (United Nations 1991). The World Health Organization estimates that only 27 percent of Haitian women between the ages of 15 and 45 years are fully vaccinated (CIAFD 1991). Large-scale surveys, however, have not traditionally captured the very deep implications of how poverty and gender work against Haitian women on almost every front. It is in the Haitian household where these bruises of poverty are most evident.

Women in the Household

Women almost always perform the array of household duties that men expect of them, not necessarily out of love but to earn their keep. For women, relationships with men may provide a trickle of cash, but they also carry high hidden costs and burdens. The physical effects of women's tasks—generating income; maintaining the house in clean and working order; washing and ironing clothes; finding, preparing, and providing food; caring for the young; and typically tending to extended kin—are heavy and are invariably concentrated during women's childbearing years (cf. Kabeer 1994; Maine et al. 1987).

Almost always there is an implicit understanding that at some time, a child must be produced if the union is to maintain itself. When resources are dangerously low, men can easily enter into women's lives, providing tiny amounts of cash. Some emergency costs might also be covered, depending on what new partners can bring to a relationship, but in most cases women said new partners helped them manage basic food costs and rent. Subsequently, men exercise their "right" to demand a child. And how can women refuse? Bearing children is often the only way, women claim, they can *kole yon nèg* (keep a man).

"As long as you're menstruating, you just keep on having children. This is how you keep a man," says Sylvia, forty-eight years old, with twelve children ranging in age from two to eighteen years. She runs a small coffee roasting business in her yard, which in Cité Soleil means just outside her front porch. Her home, which houses thirteen people, has only two rooms. The house always smells of charcoal, combined with sweet, burned coffee. Sylvia is short and thin; her shift barely hangs on her frame. She complains that the stress of life is wearing her down. Her face is weathered, and her eyes are bloodshot from regular exposure to smoke. Not only is childbearing a woman's prerogative, but it is an ideal that men encourage and expect, and women accept. Sylvia sums it up, "*si ou pa bay li, li p ap bay ou*" (if you don't give [children and to a lesser degree, sex] to him, he doesn't give [money] to you). After a sigh that leaves her looking weary, she adds, "and sometimes even if you do give, you lose anyhow. Life is hard."

Keeping a household economically viable means that pressure for both genders to make ends meet is enormous. But a close-up look at the household shows how, ultimately, discrimination falls more heavily on women's shoulders. On a daily basis, food, income allocation, and domestic violence are three areas where women are mistreated. It is in this sense that the gendered contracts are replete with discrimination. Kabeer (1994) warns that treating the household as an altruistic decision-making unit is far from the reality in households around the world, even where contracts are set. Power inside a household, defined here as control over resources, is heavily weighted in favor of men. All of the men and women, in every interview conducted in this community, resolutely agreed that men have more power than women. Lowenthal's (1984:44) findings in rural Haiti corroborate those found in Cité Soleil: "In co-residential unions, male power is reputed to be virtually limitless. Men tell their wives, they don't ask. This seigniorial privilege for the *mèt lakou* (literally, master of the household) is continuously claimed by men and, surprisingly, often upheld by women."

Countrywide, hunger and related malnutrition are considered among the most pressing problems. All but two of the women interviewed cited malnutrition (*maladi grangou*, or "hunger sickness") as one of the three most common "ailments" likely to strike them. Women are required to feed their husbands and children before they eat themselves, and "sometimes, they only smell the food" (Aristide 1994). If a woman fails to produce a meal, then she is vulnerable to verbal and physical assault. For women, especially those with children, the purchase and preparation of food is the most consuming issue in their lives. Persistent hunger means that Haitian women suffer from "maternal depletion syndrome," a term used to describe poor maternal health resulting from insufficient food. The Food and Agricultural Organization's (FAO) estimates show that 62 percent of the population were undernourished in the 1996–1998 period, constituting only a small decline from the early 1990s (FAO 2001). Although few gender-specific data are available, it is estimated that women suffer considerably more than men in this respect since hunger, coupled with closely spaced and frequent childbearing, also results in high rates of low birth weight (CIAFD 1991).

How gender interacts with economic factors is central to understanding the ways in which "being a mother [is] the most important factor disposing women to poverty" (Bruce et al. 1995). Hoddinot (cited in Kabeer 1994:104) presents data from the Ivory Coast that concurs with what has been found in Haiti: A higher proportion of women's income compared to men's is spent on goods for children and collective household consumption. Numerous women indicated that it was a man's role to *bay lajan* (give money) for general maintenance of the household but, as previously noted, few can or do. None of the women interviewed felt that men gave up everything they earned, when they actually found jobs, because of other relationships or unions that had produced children. As one woman begrudgingly said, "He seems to have his own needs." Women, on the other hand, generally reinvest all money earned directly into the household.

A study conducted by Fass (1980:72) in urban Haiti confirms what was suggested during field interviews in Cité Soleil. Among ninety-four men interviewed, just under half (49 percent) were providing what he calls "contributed-income" to the household. Although Fass claims it was not possible to fully document the purposes of the noncontributed income, he hypothesizes that it was being spent on personal goods, gambling and lottery, repayment of debts, purchase of property, and support of previous wives, families, and girlfriends. A sample of ninety women drawn at the same time showed that 82 percent were giving 100 percent of their income for the maintenance of their households. Among the 18 percent of women who were contributing less than 100 percent, 2 percent were temporary residents saving to lease their own homes, and 5 percent were sending money to their families and children in other parts of the country.

Sitting in a small marketing chair close to the ground, Dedette throws her arms in the air as she speaks, even though there is a small child sucking on her tired breast. "What do we expect of men?" she asks, with another wide gesture, she points to her shoeless feet and says, "*anyen menm*" (nothing at all). She adds, "From the moment men suspect you have money, they are at your feet like a dog, begging. But, the moment they suspect that they should provide you with one-half gourde (US$0.04), [it] comes with a slap."

Vulnerability and Violence

Around the world domestic violence is a poorly documented phenomenon, though data are increasingly demonstrating the range and extent of gender-based abuse experienced by women (Heise et al. 1994; Heise et al. 1995). At the household level, violence is spurred by conflicts over resource distribution or because men believe women do not fulfill their domestic duties. In case after case, women cited their partners for beating them for not washing or cooking, or even making something that wasn't "tasty." Women in Cité Soleil also reported they are frequently beaten for refusing sex. All the women in the community sample had been beaten at some point in their lives, and the majority on a regular basis (cf. George, cited in Heise et al. 1995:14). However, violence comes in different degrees. As a report on the topic noted, "If a man leaves a woman with two or three kids, it can be more difficult for her than if she is beaten and the next day gets 50 cents from him. [For many women] the beating is not defined as violence because it's worse to be without a source of economic support" (Shauna Swiss, personal communication 1996). Laws in Haiti reflect the reluctance of the legal system to interfere with male privilege in the home. The criminal code excuses a husband who murders his wife or her partner upon catching them in the act of adultery in his home, but a wife who kills her husband under similar circumstances is not excused.

During interviews, I discovered that violence between Haitian men and women often begins during the courtship stage, before household resources are even an issue.[6] Women tended to be younger than men during the first sexual encounter, making them more vulnerable. Twenty-one of the thirty women interviewed in Cité Soleil were forced—punched, beaten, and in one case gagged—during their first sexual encounters. Heise et al. (1995), analyzing sexuality in a gender framework from around the world, note that conditions surrounding sexual initiation are particularly important in shaping subsequent attitudes and behavior, including long-term reproductive and health outcomes. Related to the psychological implications of violence is the biological reality worldwide: Women's susceptibility to risk of infection from HIV/AIDS and other STIs is four times that of men (Gayle 2003). Studies have shown that for women, coerced sex increases the risk of micro lesions, which increase the likelihood of viral transmission. In Haiti, the lexicon men use to describe the sexual act speaks to the extent of the association with violence: *kraze yon fanm* (to crush, demolish, or break a woman), *frape* (to hit or hurl), *sakaje* (to sack or plunder), and *voye bwa tèt kale* (to club non-stop) (Adrien and Cayemittes 1991:87). Men in Cité Soleil added to this list: *chire* (to rip) and *koupe* (to cut).

Earning Their Keep: Women and Work

Nationally, women's participation in the economy, mostly as micro entrepreneurs, is comparatively high, 54 percent, as compared to the averages in both less developed countries (23 percent) and developed countries (27 percent) (UNICEF 1994a). However, women are over-represented in the lowest-paid informal sector (77 percent) while vastly under-represented in the professional private sectors (11 percent) and public sector (4 percent) (Neptune-Anglade 1995). All of the women in this study said that if they could, they would choose to live and work on their own. But few can afford to do so for extended periods without the cash inputs that men can (or promise to) deliver. Options for work and survival in Haiti are poor. The majority of women interviewed (89 percent) make up part of Haiti's vibrant informal sector of home-based businesses and market activities. For women in the informal sector, however, surviving implies great risks and huge costs.

Mimose, forty-one years old, had five children; the youngest was just learning to walk. She had been a seamstress most of her adult life and had handmade patterns, cut from butcher paper, strewn around the front room of her home. Piles of sewn and half-sewn clothes were packed into corners and on every available surface. She was wearing one of her creations—a blouse and skirt made from what looked like a drapery that once hung in a living room in the United States. Most of her clients, she says, can't afford to pay for the things they have ordered. She'll often barter food for a hand-tailored garment. She was sewing from her pedal-operated Singer machine as she talked to me, pausing frequently to describe things. When she bit the thread to cut it, she did so as close to the fabric as possible. She looked up and said: "Thread costs," anticipating my question. She nets, in a good week, US$4 for her labor. I asked if this was enough to survive. She smiled, shrugged her shoulders and said, "Hmmm. You know US$4 is not enough, but somehow we manage. We [neighbors] help each other out and we survive the pain of hunger. But I worry about my children; I have no money to send them to school."

Overall, women claim that work in the informal sector is more secure and so is more favored than work in the formal sector, because they are dependent only on themselves. All vendors hope they will break the ceiling of their earning power and become entirely self-sufficient so as to sever their dependence on men. In the words of Valerie, a market woman, "If you're good at marketing you don't need a partner. Money offers us greater freedom from dependence on men. If we had the strength, we would have a market just for women. We would not need men. The men in Haiti don't do anything. They just take us aside, have sex with us and beat us. Women are stuck inside, with the children, six naked ones hanging off their breasts, while the men sit outside together, playing games all day."

However, working as a seamstress, a one-woman restaurant, or as a vendor of plastic wares, vegetables, or locally processed peanut butter or coffee requires significant labor and capital investment. The labor required for the production of consumables, like peanut butter or coffee, is highly intensive. Peanut butter, for instance, requires the bulk purchase of raw peanuts, followed by the roasting, shelling, and removal of the coat of the peanut. Once these tasks are completed, peanuts must be ground, usually in a handheld grinder that requires a fee to use. The sale of peanut butter is usually accompanied by bread or dried cassava wafers (another investment). Working conditions, in terms of sheer physical labor, are arduous. "It's no small work to rise out of bed, your body aching from the day before, lifting that heavy load onto your head with the sun beating down as you walk toward the market," says one informant. Buying supplies in bulk is an option, but credit is available only at prohibitively high prices. At the time, lenders were charging up to 50 percent interest per month. Two hundred Haitian gourdes borrowed in June required double the sum (Hg 400) as repayment a month later. Market women are also taxed for use of market stalls in both enclosed and open market areas.[7]

A job in the formal sector, primarily in the industrial parks that surround the outskirts of Port-au-Prince, is even riskier for women. Women who look for factory jobs, either on site or at home on consignment, leave around 6:00 a.m. to stand outside the factory gates. Most wait in the unrelenting sun until at least noon before they are usually brusquely told by a factory representative that all the jobs have been taken. According to USAID, the formal sector was created specifically with women in mind because of women's "dexterity" and "patience" (NLC 1993). The labor-intensive assembly industries, which transform semifinished imported materials into finished products for export, offered Hg 15 a day or approximately US$1.00 a day. After the democratic elections in 1990, President Aristide petitioned within the business community to raise the minimum wage from Hg 15 a day to Hg 25 a day, but his proposal was adamantly rejected. After the coup d'état, among the few factories still functioning, wages fell even lower than the minimum requirement. With the reinstallment of the democratic government in 1994, the minimum wage increased to Hg 36 a day (US$2.40), a rate lower than what it was previously, due to inflation. Many women employed in factories indicated that they have not received any pay increases. In some cases, floor managers simply doubled the quantity of goods required for production in order for employees to earn the new wage (Libète 1995b:2).

Even this daily wage is quickly diminished by hidden costs of being employed in this sector: Hg 6 (approximately US$0.40) for transportation to and from work and Hg 5 (approximately US$0.34) to eat during the thirty-minute break granted mid-shift during a 6:30 a.m. to 3:30 p.m. workday. At the end of the day, income is approximately Hg 4 or US$0.27. Overtime, when actually paid out, pays one gourde (approximately US$0.07) per hour.[8]

Harassment and poor working conditions were, and continue to be, common on the factory floor. Several women told me that employees were supposed to be paid biweekly, though factory managers would often skip payroll without explanation. Employees had no recourse and often quit, since work without pay devastated the household. Several women also reported gendered abuses, in the form of rape and sexual coercion. Some women were obliged to engage in sexual relations with foremen and floor managers to get a job or keep it. Lack of resources and the dire need to remain part of the work force required some women to submit to this sexual abuse inside factories. Of thirty women from Cité Soleil who had formerly held jobs in the formal industrial sector, five reported that they were forced into sexual relations.

When Reality Hits Home:
Gender, State-Sponsored Violence, and Sex

Life has always been exhausting and rough in Cité Soleil. Respondents would often remind me of the everyday risk by saying, *se sou kont Bondyè ou ye* (you're on God's payroll). Following the coup d'état of 1991, thousands of people in Cité Soleil deserted their homes in fear of their lives. In a study completed during the post–coup d'état months, Lerebours and Canez (1992) found that over 37 percent of the population had migrated out of Cité Soleil and 65 percent of this transient population did so for economic and political reasons. Primarily, women and their children were left behind, since women—even under the gun of political terror—were expected to maintain the family unit at any cost. Here, the gendered experiences of violence dominated; the gendering effects of this "dislocation" were profound (cf. Setel 1999).

Although Haitian feminists had long been addressing violence against women as an issue of serious concern, as a "woman's issue" it spurred little public debate. The first time this violence against women was overtly discussed in the common press was when it hit epidemic proportions during the coup d'état era (Aristide 1994; François 1995; Greene 1994; Hamilton-Phelan 1994; Nifong 1994; Racine 1994). With fewer men in the community, women were exceedingly vulnerable. Some men did live in Cité Soleil (many were those fleeing rural Haiti, where repression was also rampant), but they would hide inside the small, dark households for weeks on end. Women who were hiding men noted a marked increase in domestic violence. Most of the violence, however, was state-sponsored and committed by the same military and paramilitary forces that had previously targeted politically active men.

Attacks on women-headed households at night were frequent; women were beaten and raped by the military and paramilitary at an extreme rate (Bell 1995;

Hamilton-Phelan 1994; Kennedy and Williams 1995). In almost all of the cases I identified, women had committed no crime other than being the spouse or sister of a political activist. Others were simply victims of wanton sexual crimes perpetrated by political thugs. A nurse who worked closely with the poor gave the following account: "Women suffered enormously in the three years following the coup d'état. They [military and paramilitary] raped them, they stuffed rifles up their vaginas and shot them, and pregnant women were beaten by the *chèf seksyon* until they aborted the children in their wombs."

Violence against women during the coup had no limits. One woman told me that she was forced at gunpoint to rape her son—and this was later discovered to be a common torture tactic. These crimes extended to daughters as well. An early-morning radio report alleged that groups of young girls ages ten through fourteen were being kidnapped from poor neighborhoods and sold into prostitution rings in the Dominican Republic.[9] This state-sponsored violence in Haiti was severe and received national attention from myriad international human rights organizations (MICIVIH 1995; Bell 2001).

Apart from the direct harm inflicted on female victims of these crimes, the strains that women in general endured under such volatile political and economic conditions were considerable. With President Clinton's backing, on June 23, 1993, the UN imposed a worldwide oil, arms, and financial embargo on Haiti. The embargo was meant to force the military junta from power, but many countries, including the United States, continued to trade with Haiti, and the sanctions were never enforced (NACLA 1994). The main effect was that the poor starved. The cost of food products quadrupled, and feeding a family was nearly impossible. Children chewed on twigs and roots; and mothers filled their babies' bellies with sugar cane water when there was no cash. In order to survive, women were forced to sell whatever commodities they had—sometimes it was three mangoes, or a tiny pile of charcoal. Over a period of about four months I watched many women sell nearly every possession they owned: chairs, bed, pots, and pans. Sex and reproduction, always key to survival in the Haitian context, took on exaggerated meaning.

Survival in the Market: Sex as a Commodity

Without work, and even when there was work in an increasingly weakened economy, most women in Cité Soleil who practiced serial monogamy had one of two poor choices when confronted with survival. The first "choice" was that women could hold out, and one-third of those interviewed did, with the hope that their primary partner would one day return to the household, land a job, and bring home cash. If a woman continued to provide her partner—or even a friend of his, hiding in his stead—with basic domestic needs, then she remained in the coveted primary relationship with the expectation of one day being rewarded with money for fulfillment of their conjugal contract.

Two-thirds of the sample were women who opted for the second "choice," a choice with equally little power behind it. These women were keenly aware of their partners' absence or inability to produce cash, affections, or security, so they opted out of the existing relationship to join the ranks of female-headed households. Statistics for this sample of women reflect the trend in Cité Soleil where, according to the clinic's head doctor, approximately 60 percent of all households in Cité Soleil were female-headed (personal communication, Despagne 1993).[10] Under these circumstances the political economy of Haiti clearly penetrated the gender system and put women at a now more deadly disadvantage than ever.

Structural forces, made heavier by the embargo, produced an almost immediate blow to the women left behind. Within days of the embargo, women's most important source of daily income, the informal market sector, turned moribund. Not only were imports and exports prohibited, but without access to gasoline, the internal movement of produce from the countryside to the city came to a screeching halt. For women desperate for cash, sex became one of the few existing viable market assets: US$1.75 for an unprotected encounter, enough to buy three small oranges or one small can of evaporated milk, or US$5.00 for an encounter with a virgin. Women ventured into middle-class neighborhoods to sell their bodies. The actual financial value of sexual exchanges at the time was extremely low, though vital for all, since the economic rewards, when pooled, could help tide starving families over for a few days.

Sex for cash exchanges, performed outside the conjugal relationship and most commonly by women in female-headed households, became more common. According to those interviewed, the nature of these paid sexual exchanges is considered distinctly different from work of a *bouzen* or woman who performs sexual transactions as a profession. Women interviewed in this study did not work in brothels, nor did they get dressed and go to town. Sexual exchanges were appropriately called *travay* (work). Men—knowing women were in desperate circumstances—would often pass by the house and inquire somewhat discreetly about sexual opportunities. Sometimes these men were acquaintances, though often they were strangers. Of the three women who described these episodes, not one indicated they used condoms. When asked why not, all three said the exact same words: *nou pa gen dwa* (we don't have the right).

Women's accounts of sex for cash were filled with humiliation. During the course of the interviews when the subject of "work" came up, the dialogue would lose its intensity. Women would bite their lips and look away, turning their heads, as if to hold back tears. Yvonne was one of these women. She was the mother of twin girls. Her partner, persecuted by the military, left on an illegal boat with promises of sending cash once he found a job *lòt bò lamè*—on the other side of the ocean (i.e., Miami). It had been over a year since he left, and Yvonne assumed he drowned, though there was no clear proof of this. The US$1.75 she made for each "work" episode was only enough to fill part of a medical prescription.

She was coughing up blood while we spoke. She described the sexual encounter as "numbing," since she rarely knew the men that paid her for these transactions. Sometimes, she told me, these men would hit her and force her on the cement floor of her house. After divulging the uncomfortable details of her sexual encounters, there was a long silence. She ended it, when neither of us knew what to say, with this: *nou pa merite sa* (we don't deserve this).

These desperate sexual encounters meant that all women and men in this community were at increased health risk. The possibility of contracting sexually transmitted infections (STIs) was a significant reproductive health risk during the post–coup d'état era, though it was hard to determine if STIs were on the rise, since no one knew the prevalence before the coup. However, in a pilot study conducted in Cité Soleil during 1993, STI prevalence among women (men were not included in the study) was reported to be 60 percent (CDS 1993). The majority of these diseases went untreated for lack of proper diagnosis, lack of money to purchase medications, and failure to inform patients' partners. All of the women interviewed indicated that the gender inequalities that pervade relationships contribute significantly to women's failure to inform their partners of risk. HIV/AIDS is a risk for men, women, and the children born to them. An HIV study showed that 10.5 percent of sexually active women in Cité Soleil (between the ages of 15 and 45) were seropositive (Brutus 1989).

While sexual survival strategies, coupled with a low use of condoms, is dangerous for both men and women, "safe sex" messages are insufficient. A nurse working in the community insists that this risk be analyzed within a gendered perspective. "If women are dying from childbirth and . . . AIDS, it is because they cannot negotiate with men." Over the decade of fieldwork, however, I met very few women whose partners would consent to using condoms. Men, on the other hand, indicated that indeed they do use condoms sporadically and almost always with partners outside their primary relationship. The same men generally concurred that they do not use condoms in their primary relationships (because as one man said, "she would suspect me"), thus placing their primary partners in grave danger of contracting a STI. In Cange, Haiti, the prevalence of forced sex in a population accessing services at a women's health project was 54 percent. "This significant prevalence of forced sex is sadly not surprising, given the steep grade of gender inequality that exists in Haiti" (Smith Fawzi et al. 2005:684).

In addition to the risk of sexually transmitted infections and violence, forced and unprotected sexual encounters also impact unwanted fertility and the risk of related mortality. When gender inequality interacts with poverty, women's health risks increase yet again. Confirming this, worldwide, the highest maternal mortality rates (MMRs) are all in Africa and in rank order, Rwanda, Sierra Leone, Burundi, Ethiopia, Somalia, Chad, Sudan, Burkina Faso, Equatorial Guinea, Angola, and Kenya. In all, there are twenty two countries in sub-Saharan Africa with MMRs of 1,000 or higher. Here too, Haiti stands as a hemispheric outlier, being the only country outside of the African continent with a value in excess of 1,000 (UNFPA 2001). At the time my fieldwork was being conducted, maternal mortality rates in Port-au-Prince increased from an average 520/100,000, already the highest in the hemisphere, to 1,110/100,000.[11]

During the same time period, SOFA (*Solidaritè Fanm Ayisyen*), a women's organization based in Port-au-Prince, cited an increase in mismanaged abortions conducted by nonphysicians under appalling conditions. During one two-week period in May 1993, the University of Haiti's General Hospital in Port-au-Prince admitted seventeen young women between the ages of fourteen and twenty five who were infected after undergoing abortions. One died, and doctors had to remove the wombs of two others (Chanel 1993). During the coup d'état era, the potential burden of a child was so overwhelming that when abortions or family planning were not options, some even resorted to deserting their babies. In January of 1994, I witnessed two tiny babies—one dead with its hands wrapped in cord and another barely breathing, deserted on the main avenue of Cité Soleil.

Where Power Reigns and Gender Shifts

Typically, where patriarchy reigns, gender inequality is explained in economic terms (Correa 2000). But a resource-based approach, focusing simply on men's economic power over women, falls short of explaining all the dynamics that define gender systems. In the realm of sex and reproduction, power is spread unevenly across the social and cultural grid. These dynamics are also constantly in flux. Capturing the extent to which reproduction influences people's lives is critical to understanding what public health interventions might work best.

In Haiti, men and women are challenged to enact very different, though intimately related, survival strategies. In this community, options are few and for most people *zanmi ede zanmi* (friends help friends) to survive, with survival taking on many forms. Though the perceptions of both genders continue to lean, however helplessly, toward the cultural ideal (a man who provides for and protects his wife for the sake of his entire household, and a woman who serves as a healthy and capable mother and partner in her prescribed domestic role), harsh reality dictates otherwise. Parenthood and the obligations these roles demand have taken on increasingly rough contours. Children are clearly the products of the tenuous gender relations that define life among the poor in urban Haiti.

Lock and Kaufert (1988) identify selective reproductive strategies—or pragmatism—pursued by women, including those that challenge dominant ideologies, as a form of resistance. Building on this and in the context of what the authors call "changing patterns of constraint" in people's lives, pragmatism here is expanded to include the lives of men. Haitians, when in limited social and economic contexts, call on sexuality and reproduction as a means of survival. In Cité Soleil, the gender system (Correa 2000; Rubin 1975), as articulated by both women and men, is rapidly shifting under heavy economic, social, and political pressures.

In these shifts, power is expressed in multiple ways: through male identity and machismo, through women's calculated reproductive decisions, and, in its most extreme form, through violence in the household and community. These dynamics, set against a backdrop of ongoing structural violence, are critical determinants of reproductive health and outcomes in Haiti.

For men in Cité Soleil, the collapse of the Haitian economy and high rates of unemployment have ensured drastically reduced economic power. With little currency and denied sources of self-esteem through productive work, men are suffering from emasculation. This, compounded by the ongoing terror of repressive politics, has diminished the status of Haitian men in their own eyes, as well as women's, in the family and in the community. Devoid of steady financial resources and unable to stand up to the violence perpetrated in their communities by the state, men simply cannot act responsibly toward women and their children. Although men try to provide sporadic incomes as economic support for women, women generally lose in the long term because inevitably they must produce a child (Lowenthal 1984).

In the face of these grim prospects, men appear to be clinging even more doggedly to their only power—that over women. The higher cost of sex with a virgin, even at a time when people weren't eating for days during the embargo, is emblematic of what men would pay to exert and express their power via their sexuality. Sex in Cité Soleil is also regulated through violence and, in many ways, this represents the "quintessential, testosteronic expression of male entitlement" (Landes, cited in Altman 2001:6). Altman's work on the globalization of sex suggests that sexual violence is a growing part of the current global disorder. Rape, Altman contends, is a way of "preserving tradition" and in the case of Haitian men, who are fast losing all of their traditional roles in society, this makes unfortunate sense. It is clear, too, that through acts of violence and rape, men are responding to the structural systems—both political and economic—that control them. Violence in its many forms is a way of reasserting the eroding male identity.

Women's power is often confined to specific realms: the household, motherhood, and sexuality. In Cité Soleil, women use what power they have to counteract existing inequalities in the gender system. When women ask men, *sa ou pote pou mwen?* (what do you have for me?), they are using sex for economic leverage. Here, if even for a brief moment, they have the upper hand. The price of virginal sexual encounters was ultimately set by women, thus reflecting some form of control. Yet, sex is usually embedded in a network of power relations and is, at least for women, more often based on obligation, largely to children. In the end, women in Cité Soleil will do just about anything to ensure that their children survive, typically under conditions where they are generally unable to negotiate all of the terms of their relationships. Structural forces also have clear impacts on women's reproductive health. Zapata et al. (1992) notes that the presence of police and military, undercover police activity, demonstrations—all common in

Cité Soleil—are factors that contributed to a fivefold increase in poor pregnancy outcomes in Chile. In simple biological terms, then, for women sex and reproduction carry considerably more dangers than for men—disease, unwanted fertility, and severe obstetric complications.

Men, Women, Use Family Planning!

The family planning slogan for the Ministry of Health in the late 1980s, *Mesye, Danm Fè Planing!* (Men, Women, Use Family Planning!) was once ubiquitous in the capital: on billboards, clinic doors, and in waiting rooms. And yet, saddled with this lack of control and the dire reproductive health consequences that result from promiscuity and procreation, why do Haitians, both men and women, not opt for family planning? It seems that family planning would be the easiest way to avoid the short-term risks of STIs and the long-term costs of maternal morbidity or of bearing a child. The answer, from this gendered perspective, is obviously complex, bound up in both the political economy and the culture of reproduction in Haiti.

Family planning, it is often argued, offers people a distinct form of empowerment by allowing women and men access to methods of fertility regulation and more control over their bodies. Nerlande, a former contraceptive user with five children, now heads her own household and claims celibacy. She differs with this thinking. Dressed in a blouse that once belonged to a gas station attendant named Jimmy in the United States and a straight skirt that covers her pencil-thin legs, she was kind and informative during our interviews. When family planning was discussed, her demeanor changed to one of anger. For Nerlande, clinic visits equated to long waits and troublesome side effects that led to her partner's disapproval—so much so that he left her for not "producing." During the interview she grew frustrated with the "but whys?" that rolled from my tongue. Exasperated, she threw her hands up, trying to end the long interview and said, "Don't you understand? I stopped using *planing*, because it controlled me!" Women's use or resistance to the use of family planning is reflected in the many gender inequities that define their lives. This degree of gender inequality, compounded by the deep poverty experienced by women in Haiti, puts women at significant risk of HIV infection and other STDs as well as unwanted fertility (Farmer, Connors, and Simmons, 1997). In Cité Soleil, these inequalities are reinforced by men's understanding of family planning.

Family Planning by Gender

Men's opinions about family planning were also tied to notions of power and control. Many men in this community did not want their female partners to use family planning because it was perceived as giving women the power to control their reproductive health, a central aspect of their lives. Several men told me, using similar words, that family planning gives women "more [sexual] freedom than they need." No matter how slight, this autonomy threatened prevailing power relationships between men and women.[12]

Women were clear in explaining how using family planning was a loaded issue. Women who used family planning were regularly vulnerable to humiliation and violence. For women, fear or lack of negotiating power figured prominently in the discourse, particularly because if they insisted on using contraception they ran the risk of losing their partner's support. Janine was dressed in a tight black skirt and a large T-shirt with a "Notre Dame University—Fighting Irish" emblem on it. She had been going to the clinic for years and used Depo-Provera so that she could hide her method from her partner. She was monogamous, but was recently diagnosed with an infection. "He tells me he will not use the condom," she said. "They always give me condoms at the clinic and say, 'Now use this with your partner.' I ask him to use it; he says no. It's not a small refusal; he'll slap me when he's angry. This is why they [men] tell us that one single woman isn't suffi-cient; if I don't give, the other [woman] will."

Gladys, another clinic client, headed a household and had sexual relations with a "friend" who provided small amounts of money to her for the exchanges. Even during these types of exchanges, she explained, women simply cannot demand protection. The extent to which women understand their status, and yet can do little to change it, is poignant. "It's like I told you, if someone's behind you, wishing to make friends with you . . . Before he gives you money, you have to sleep with him, and it's during these times when children are born. Ask him to put on a condom? Hah! On the contrary, he accuses me of not trusting him, which effec-tively means that he refuses to use a condom. *Women are obliged to be exploited*" (my emphasis).

Tied up in men's opposition to family planning, as a means of women's lib-eration, is the way that modern methods were viewed as unnatural. Men claimed that modern methods *gate nati fi a* (spoils women's nature). And these arguments reflected their gendered expectations of women as both producers and repro-ducers in the domestic domain. Jean Luc, for instance, who was twenty-five years old, had fathered four children by two different women. He reiterated what men said to me again and again: "Women are made for having children. Why block what nature has intended? Besides, when a woman starts using *planing* it only gives her more problems. They have allergies to it, they get sick and then well, when a woman suffers, so do we because who will manage the household?"

Another male informant corroborated. "That three-month shot [Depo-Provera] and five-year method [Norplant], they take away a woman's period. Women must have their periods. When a woman doesn't have her period, she's not made for love; and when she's not made for love, she can't have children. That's not good."

Women's rationale against family planning was equally and persuasively linked not only to men's expectations of women but to women's expectations of themselves, defined by men's gendered preferences. Among former users and nonusers, when asked reasons for not using modern methods of birth control, the curt and simple reply, *mari mwen pa vle* (my husband doesn't want it), was common. But further discussion always led to countless examples of how women, too, claimed that family planning gate nati fi a. "Spoiled nature" for women referred to a host of physically debilitating symptoms that often accompany family planning use, including irregular bleeding, increased discharge, and general weakness. "It's not that we want to have many children. The poor are poor, and more children make life more difficult. But *planing* spoils the nature of the woman. This is what makes family planning bad; your partner will leave you with the house full of children and he'll look for another woman. If you are 'spoiled,' he doesn't want you. This is the main reason women don't want to use family planning."

The spoiled nature of women has commonly been interpreted by outside observers simply as a "folk belief." But the term has much broader gender-infused interpretations. It is packed with meaning in terms of women's prescribed role in sex. Any number of side effects, such as *bouboun dlo* (watery vagina—essentially a well-lubricated vagina or one with abnormal discharge), according to Lowenthal (1984) render women sexually undesirable and are believed to cause a spoiled nature. Significantly, as Yvonne, a former user, later clarified, these are the conditions of "frivolous" women, conditions that do not match those of an upstanding female partner or mother.

Many of the men interviewed had used family planning—exclusively condoms—but usually with casual partners. When I asked why, they were always quick to respond: *SIDA manje nou* (AIDS is killing us), and this was often followed by a list of other sexually transmitted infections they knew they could catch. Even though condom use was increasingly widespread over the ten years of fieldwork, it was reported as sporadic. Several men told me, laughing, that they would use condoms, but often followed with a statement "if I remember." Men do not like the way condoms feel and find them cumbersome. Many men told me they prefer a dry vaginal environment during intercourse. When I expressed this to some of the experts at USAID, as well as in the clinic, it was called a "cultural barrier" and left at that. The condoms offered at the Cité Soleil clinic were the lubricated variety and for years efforts to change this type were all for naught. Since then, the purportedly successful social marketing campaign for condom use has made access easier and has apparently enhanced their appeal for men. Social marketing, a technique used in public health circles, aims to "reach" one or a number of target groups to initiate and effect changes in their ideas and behavior. Population Services International/AIDSMark, an organization working in Haiti, carried out a highly successful condom marketing initiative there. The "Pantè" (panther) condom was widely promoted and sold locally for less than 20 percent of the price of popular commercial condom brands. Pantè sales have increased steadily since the condom's introduction in 1992.

Experts confirm that increased condom use has appeared to have slowed the number of AIDS cases in Haiti (Chanel 1997).

Although some men do understand the benefits of family planning, primarily for spacing children, they typically abdicate responsibility for both limiting the numbers of children they sire and for using contraceptives themselves. There are some women (none whom I interviewed but some whom I met) who have partners who cooperate in their efforts to control their fertility. But these women are the exceptions. Generally women were on their own. Among the community sample of women (divided among contraceptive users, former users, and nonusers), current users did not have overwhelming support from their partners. Eight of the ten users kept their family planning decisions to themselves and did not share this information with either their close friends or their partners.

From a gendered perspective, repeated short-term unions forbid long-term contraceptive use. Accepting and continuing with a family planning method assumes that women can afford not to have children, but our journey into Haitian households reveals the contrary. Even when women want to avoid the risk of a STI or pregnancy, rarely are they in positions to negotiate with their partners—in their own words, they simply "don't have the right." As individuals, women and men do not have the power to countervail the cultural and economic forces that tell them not to use contraceptives. This lack of choice is a serious violation of everyone's rights, but particularly women's. A friend from Cité Soleil framed it in the rawest terms possible when she recounted a now popular saying: *Si ou sere koko, w ap manje kaka* (If you close your vagina, you'll eat shit).

Analyzing reproduction within the PEF framework provides the depth needed to demonstrate how gender concepts and relations should play a prominent role in development policy and practice, particularly as it relates to reproductive health. Although gender as a concept now infuses the family planning rhetoric, moving it into the realm of actual interventions is critical. Understanding survival by gender is key to designing effective family planning programs, and yet little attention has been paid to these loaded gendered arenas.

In the next chapter, I move from the privacy of the household into the more public, clinic setting. I observe women who feel empowered enough to use family planning as they confront and challenge the medicalization of their reproduction. I show how these "pragmatic" women negotiate their power—or lose what little they have—in the heart of the biomedical setting.

4

The Family Planning Center

A Clinic in Conflict

Perhaps the most critical transaction of all in family planning programs is that between the program and the client, for all others ultimately revolve around that nexus. If this transaction fails, the program will fail with it.

–Donald Warwick, Bitter Pills

There had been no electricity in Haiti for month-long stretches during the embargo of 1994; March 30 was no exception. Inside the clinic it was a typical afternoon: hot, sticky, and very still. The staff sat on their metal folding chairs, staring blankly, waiting for the doctors to arrive. The nurse, preparing cotton balls and alcohol, exclaimed that it was too hot to move. Nine women from the community, referred to by the staff as *kliyan* (clients), sat on hard wooden benches in the waiting room. Some were dressed in clothes reserved for Sunday mass and doctor's visits. Others were too poor and wore rags. All came to the clinic for more pills, another Depo-Provera shot, or relief from irregular bleeding or itching and burning "down there." Each hoped that the doctor would allay her discomfort.

The doctors saw the clients upstairs. The two Haitian doctors were tall and heavy by national standards. They always looked neat and cool when they arrived in their crisp clothing and inevitably they, too, commented on how hot the clinic was. They spoke impeccable French. Their Creole, unlike that of the poor women who attend the clinic, was studded with French phrases, confirming that they were both urban-born and educated. One of the doctors marked his clients' charts with a fancy gold pen. Work in Cité Soleil, while uncomfortable and often bothersome, paid well. Haitian doctors are frustrated by a consistent lack of supplies and little credit for the work they do. They are clearly bored, repeating the same instructions for several hours each afternoon. Both of the doctors held jobs in other medical practices, and the job in Cité Soleil was really only for the extra cash it brought. Doctors working for the Centers for Health and Development (CDS, its French acronym) were compensated for their "hardship posts."

International organizations, especially USAID, inflate salaries for third-world professionals, in the case of Haiti, to nearly three times that of a doctor working in a clinic of the Ministry of Health. In addition, doctors can commute from the world of the poor (Cité Soleil) to the world of the elite in less than thirty minutes. And there are far worse options, such as working in rural Haiti (personal correspondence, Paul Farmer 2003).

The two examining rooms were small and sparse. The rooms were filled with the din from Route Nationale #1, Haiti's major thoroughfare. Sometimes when the semis honked, it was so loud that both the doctor and client winced. The stifling rooms were coated with a layer of dust that seeped in through the window slats. Since electricity is not a constant on Cité Soleil's grid, the old examining lamps were pushed into the corner. For light, the doctors cranked open the slatted windows, positioning the rays of sunlight on their clients' groins.

I was poised in my anthropologist-researcher role: observation form in hand, a tape recorder perched on the desk. Conversations were recorded and actions noted during each doctor-patient interaction observed. An interaction, or encounter, in this study was defined as beginning when the client entered the doctor's office and ending when she left. Individual family planning clients shuffled in and out of the doctors' rooms, sometimes as many as sixty per doctor every afternoon.

Yvonne entered with some hesitancy. She was twenty-four years old, unemployed, and the reproductive history scribbled on her chart indicated she had four children. She had come to the clinic for more birth control pills. She stood nervously clutching her big vinyl purse.

DOCTOR: Enter! Have you had your period?

CLIENT: Yes.

D: When did it come?

C: It comes every twenty-eight days.

D: It came today?

C: No, it hasn't come yet.

D: Because—you were supposed to come on the 16th, and you didn't come.

C: I couldn't come, I was busy that day.

D: But if you don't have your period, I can't give you the pills.

C: But it will come anyhow.

D: It's not an affair of waiting, *madame*. It must be here for me to give you the pills. It's been fourteen days since you have taken the pills, and where is your period?

C: I took them. It was two packets of pills that you gave me.

D: It wasn't two packets. It was only one, *madame*.

C: Well, maybe you didn't mark it. I took two. I still had pills. That's why I didn't come earlier.

D: (*Mumbling to himself*) She took one packet in January, one packet in February, I marked it.

C: I took two packets in January.

D: But if you took two packets—I'll tell you a little thing. If you took two packets in January, you should have come in early March. So where does that leave you now? On your head or what?

C: I haven't fallen. It seems like you didn't mark it, because you gave me two packets.

D: (*Throwing the chart at her*) Where do you see that? Where do you see that?

C: Then . . . (shaking, she reaches into her purse, for an empty packet).

D: Well, it's finished. For that matter—are you taking them at home? Where's the other packet? Where is it, huh? If it's two you have, huh? So, you don't have your period, you missed your appointment and you're not taking your pills. I'm giving you condoms, *madame*. When you have your period, come here again. If you don't want condoms, tell me rapidly that you're not OK with this.

C: You can give them to me.

D: When your period arrives you'll come here.

C: Yes.

D: OK.

In the last minute of the transaction, with the client still present, the doctor, exasperated, wrote on a tiny piece of paper, "*The Black Jacobins* by C.L.R. James" and slid it over to me, asking if I had read this definitive account of the Haitian Revolution of 1791–1803. I nodded yes, perplexed by the reference to the book during the encounter. He raised his finger and said, "One minute." He finished with the client and sent her from the room, then looked at me. He said,

Do you remember in the book there is a slave? Those slaves they were stupid and they lied. They could easily hold you in their lies. The slave he stole a pigeon. He put it in his shirt, and his master caught him. His master said, "You stole that pigeon!" The slave denies it, saying "I don't know how that pigeon got underneath my shirt!" And the pigeon is flapping wildly inside his shirt. Do you understand? Their mentality hasn't changed. It's the same thing with this woman: She's so stupid that—that she says she took two packets of pills, but she didn't. Oh! It's all the same! They're still stupid, they still lie and they're still slaves!

The referenced passage in *The Black Jacobins* varies slightly but significantly from this doctor's version. In the historical account, the master who accused the slave of stealing is the same man who had minutes before *sent* the slave to steal the pigeon; without warning, "the master orders him a punishment of 100 lashes to which the slave submits without a murmur" (James 1989:15). Later, when I checked a daily register of clinic data, I saw that the doctor had in fact prescribed two packets of pills for Yvonne. Like the master in the literary passage, the doctor, during his consultation, failed to admit his own mistake and punished the client for it, denying her preferred method of contraception or a reasonable alternative.

Yvonne's encounter, like the 154 others I observed, encapsulates how the doctor-client relationship is a domain where ideology—doctrine of a distinctive perspective—is reproduced. The asymmetrical relationship, including an infallible doctor and the initially challenging client who, in the end, has no choice but to agree with the accusations made against her, reflects and replicates the dominating structures that reverberate throughout Haitian society. In this way, as Waitzkin contends, "Medical encounters become micropolitical situations that reflect and support broader social relations, including social class and political-economic power" (1991:9). Treatment such as Yvonne received is not unusual in Haiti. It conforms to the society's dominant expectations about appropriate behavior toward the poor, behavior that the majority of Haitians have endured for nearly two hundred years.

Doctors generally represent a small slice of Haiti's privileged class. Clients in the clinic were primarily landless peasants who migrated to this destitute urban community for lack of other choices. To challenge what goes on during the doctor-client encounter inside the family planning clinic is, ultimately, to challenge the social conditions in Haiti, including a vast class disparity, social hierarchy and, primarily, poverty. Already bridled by their gendered experiences in the private domains of their lives, women who come to the clinic are further diminished in the clinical encounter. Focus on the social dynamics between doctors and family planning clients revealed reasons for resistance to contraceptive use that transcend traditional public health parameters. Barriers to care were often hidden within language and manner. Clinical encounters are strong reminders that "although the decision to regulate fertility involves key health considerations, it is also a social act requiring negotiating power" (Bongaarts and Bruce 1995:73). Without such power, clients simply cannot win.

The Family Planning Center

The family planning center of Cité Soleil first opened its doors in September 1983. At that time family planning was a relatively new concept to this community.

Family health surveys done in 1981 and 1983 indicated that only 6 percent of residents were using modern contraceptives (Boulos 1985). Yet the same report indicated that illegal abortions were on the rise and a "demand" existed for contraceptives, and so the family planning center opened, but not without resistance. The order of Belgian nuns, who managed food depots, schools, and several other facilities in the community, were opposed to family planning, because of the Catholic Church's position on birth control. Where one religious community obstructed, another facilitated, and eventually the Baptist Convention of Haiti offered a building that housed the family planning center.

The center has relocated twice since 1983. There was cause for celebration in July 1991, when the clinic moved to the new quarters on Route Nationale #1. The new building, both spacious and split-level, was well located next to the busiest entrance to the community. Outside the door of the clinic hung a hand-painted sign: Centre de Protection Maternelle/CDS (the Center for Maternal Protection/Centers for Health and Development). CDS leaders felt that using the terms "maternal" and "protection" was a benign way of referring to family planning without actually offending the Belgian nuns, who twelve years later remained defiantly opposed to family planning activities in this slum community. The clinic was referred to by the staff and clients who attended it as *sant planin* (planning center).

Based on an estimated 10 to 15 percent use of contraception among women of reproductive age countrywide (CHI/CDC 1991), the clinic should have been providing services for approximately 4,500 to 6,500 women. In fact, the numbers attending were considerably lower, fewer than 1,500 regular users in 1994. Fewer clients were attending than in previous years, when the family planning center was located in a nearby house in much more cramped quarters (Burton 1993). The International Planned Parenthood Federation (IPPF), the international agency that helped fund clinic activities, claimed it was "unclear" whether a lower proportion of women in Cité Soleil actually practiced family planning than the 10 to 15 percent rate reported nationally by the CDC or whether women were going elsewhere for services (Burton 1993). Either way, it was clear that services were not filling the supposed "need" in Cité Soleil. Yet more money was poured into this clinic, and IPPF reported that the cost per user in Cité Soleil was one of the highest among all the programs they funded worldwide. IPPF investigated the problem and attributed the low number of users to a declining quality of services and "in particular very poor patient/provider interaction" (Burton 1993:2).

The Social Wall: The Clinic Space as Symbolic

Although the layout of the center may seem inconsequential at first glance, its spatial context and the processes played out within it were significant. Comaroff (1985:54) emphasizes the importance of space, full of "elemental signs with hidden meanings, mediating between the sociocultural system and the experiencing subjects . . . within it." On a symbolic level, the physical space and arrangement of the clinic area reinforced, in less than subtle ways, the division of class and status within the family planning center.

The reception room was huge, though it rarely accommodated more than ten to fifteen clients at any time. Twelve brown wooden benches and random folding chairs filled the area, two small metal desks were placed in the front of the room, and a scale for weighing clients was lodged in a corner. Nothing hung on the walls. It gave the distinct message that clients should not be comfortable. Clients often succumbed to their boredom and would lie horizontally, napping, while they waited for service. Two small areas in the front room were reserved for reception and for the auxiliary nurse who would take vital signs. A television monitor, supposedly for audiovisual materials, installed in the corner of the reception room, was encased in a metal cage, though this did not stop vandals from stealing the equipment, which was never used anyway. There was air circulating, but it was the dry and very dusty air that swirled in from the noisy, speeding public transportation vehicles just outside the clinic walls. Inside, the walls were painted half green and half white, colors long since adopted by the Ministry of Health to denote a health facility.

Family planning promoters, who occupied the lowest rung in the staff hierarchy, worked both in the field and the clinic, serving as mediators, escorting clients to the center and speaking to them as they entered. The promoters were women from the community who were trained to provide education and counseling on contraceptive methods in the privacy of residents' homes in order to prepare potential clients for their visit and improve the overall quality of care. They would also escort clients to the clinic, and they often sat on the benches in the waiting room, next to clients. It was an unstated rule that such close contact with the client would be inappropriate behavior for any other staff. That the promoters were not allowed to drink water from a cooler available to all other clinic staff—even though their work in the hot sun and stifling homes was arduous—was but one indication of how promoters, too, were viewed and distanced, both physically and socially.

Just behind the reception area was the room that held patient files, appropriately located within reach of the staff that search for records. This room also housed the much-coveted water cooler. The Norplant room offered the most privacy and was the most spacious of all rooms in the clinic. Despite the sign on the door that said, "Counseling," the counseling was limited to Norplant users, who were actively recruited to encourage more women to adopt this long-term method. The nursing station was the smallest room in the center. Here, with only minimal privacy, clients received injectables, pills, condoms, and some instruction on how to use them. The nursing station also served as a social area of sorts where the nurses and auxiliaries drank colas and gossiped while they waited for the doctors, since no clinical activity occurred until they arrived.

The location of the doctors' examining rooms, upstairs and farthest from the clients' waiting area, reinforced the hierarchal social order of the clinic. The two rooms were fairly small (3 m × 3.3 m and 2.4 m × 4 m); both rooms had a desk, one chair and an examining table with stirrups and dirty sheets. The yellowing cream-colored walls were empty, except for large clumps of dust that collected in the walls' seams. In each room a small stainless steel cart held a messy array of latex medical gloves, cotton, swabs, clamps piled in an old, flimsy cardboard box, and typically empty bottles of fixant spray for cytology slides. Overhead fans, air conditioning units, fixtures for an overhead light, and a small examining light were all rendered useless because electricity was rarely supplied to the clinic. The CDS clinic director, who oversaw six family planning centers around the country, also had a private office (2.4 m × 3 m) on the upper level.

Social distancing in this clinic, reinforced by social space, ensured that clients felt like outsiders, even though the clinic was, ostensibly, there to serve them.[1] As the staff gained professional status, they were located farther and farther from the waiting room, where clients convened. In the waiting room, clients were virtually unattended and were provided with huge and hard spaces. However, in the nursing station and the doctors' examining rooms, where they received care, clients were excessively cramped both physically and socially. The cramped quarters seemed to justify doctors' and nurses' hurried, abrupt, and rude exchanges with clients. It was not uncommon to see nurses and doctors physically recoil when more destitute clients were in need of services. It was as if they were repulsive. This distancing from social inferiors by emotional and physical means has been called the "social wall" in Haitian society (Trouillot 1995a). Few can cross, let alone approach it. The layout of the clinic reinforced the social divide at every step of the clients' quest for therapy.

Filling the Mandate: Quality of Care

Services offered at the center were limited to the provision of family planning methods: oral contraceptives, Depo-Provera (three-month injectables), Norplant (a subdermal implant that provides protection for up to five years), intrauterine devices (IUDs), condoms, and foam tablets. At one point during data collection a small research study was under way to determine the prevalence of sexually transmitted infections (STIs) from a client-based sample, but such testing was by no means the norm in this clinic. At the time, clinicians were also encouraged to include breast exams as part of a client's initial screening, but again, this was not the normal protocol. These services were provided, either directly or indirectly, by a staff of nineteen people: an administrative head physician, two gynecologists, one head nurse, another nurse explicitly in charge of the Norplant

program, a receptionist/auxiliary/computer operator and her assistant, two auxiliary nurses, nine family planning promoters, and a groundskeeper.

All clinic activities were directed toward delivering quality services for women
in need of family planning. The USAID mandate at the time focused on the Quality
of Care Framework (Bruce 1989)—a framework that has since become an essential part of global population discourse (Richey 1999b). It prompts program
planners to reassess services using criteria that go beyond counting clients,
the dispensing of various family planning methods, type of visit, and so on, and
focuses instead on delivering services in a user-friendly way. The framework was
thus a boon to the feminist advocacy agenda of promoting women's rights
within the family planning setting. The principal criteria for assessing the quality of family planning programs within this framework are: choice of methods,
information given to users, technical competence of the staff, interpersonal
relations, follow-up or continuity mechanisms, and appropriateness of the services provided (Bruce 1989).

Viewing the Cité Soleil family planning center activities in terms of this
framework is instructive. Here, I will mainly focus on provider-client interactions (referred to as interpersonal relations in the framework). These interactions provide a window into other areas of quality. However, they do not provide
the sole source of information. Limiting the analysis to interactions between
doctor and patient would narrowly define the clinic experience as an isolated
dyad rather than as part of a medical institution, itself integrated into a specific,
historically constructed social and political framework (Lazarus 1988). Additional information provided by clinical procedures, staff meetings, and interviews illuminate the institutional context, shedding light on how power is
distributed throughout the health care system.

The Encounter

Several types of clients attended this clinic—current family planning users, former
users, and nonusers—and they visited for multiple reasons. When new Cité Soleil
clients passed through the doors of the clinic they proceeded to the receptionist,
who would take a short history and fill out a family planning file. Blood pressure
was checked, and an auxiliary nurse sitting nearby weighed the client. A continuing client (one who had been to the clinic before) would give her numerically
coded family planning card to the receptionist who would locate her chart. The
clients would hold their charts and sometimes receive group education on method
choice, side effects, and contraindications. The content and quality of these sessions varied considerably, depending on the interest and the family planning
promoter giving the education. Some clients slept during the presentation, others partook in animated socially and politically packed dialogue. Once this
intake process was completed and the doctors had arrived, the client was sent

upstairs with her family planning card and chart. Clients waited for their consultation on benches just outside the consultation room.

Encounters, in general, were full of conflict. One of the doctors yelled frequently, particularly when he was frustrated with women unprepared for examinations, which were a standard of care for all new clients. Many women did not know how to lie on the examining table (having never seen one before) or how to put their feet in the stirrups. This unfamiliarity appeared to agitate the doctors even more, to the point of ridiculing women. Doctors would typically deliver rapid orders in stern and loud voices, full of disdain, while women timidly and nervously undressed.

"Take off your underwear, take them off. Not your skirt, just get the underwear! Off!"

"What's the matter with you? You're cowardly, come on *madame!*"

"Why are you trembling? *Madame*, look, if you can't open [your legs], it's because you have an infection, now open."

"Put your bottom here, down! Down! Open your legs!"

"No! Put your feet here! Here! Like you're on a donkey. What's your problem, you've never been on a donkey?"

It was routine to hear patients yelling out in pain and fear during the exams. Rough treatment was the norm in this clinic.

The consultation completed, the client was then directed to go back downstairs and receive her family planning method from the nurse in the nursing station. Once she had this, she gave her file back to the receptionist. The receptionist then recorded the client's activity in a daily journal/log book and filled out a corresponding form. The client was then free to leave. Many clients would indeed leave, never to come back. A review of some of the encounters explains why.

Courtesy, Time, and Choice: Respect or Neglect?

Greetings are an implicit part of Haitian language and are very basic *politès* (politeness, kindness), expected of everyone in every setting. Yet they did not occur in the medical encounter in this clinic. Greetings of "hello" (*bonjou/bonswa*) or "how are you" (*ki jan ou ye*) were given six times in the entire sample of 154 encounters. In most encounters the doctors would merely shout out "Enter!" ordering the next client to the consultation room. The majority of encounters began like this: "When did you get your period?" "Have you seen your blood?" "How many days has your blood been flowing?" "Did your period come?" Most of the time the doctors would ask these questions without ever glancing at the clients.

Time, an important dimension of a medical encounter, is costly in Haiti. For women, time at the clinic could be spent at the market selling, or in the factory producing, or at home tending to the multiple needs of family and extended kin. All these activities are crucial to maintaining the fragile balance in a poor Haitian household. And yet the average wait before seeing the doctor in this clinic was approximately one hour and four minutes, in contrast to the average doctor's visit, which lasted approximately two minutes.[2] The consultation presented at this chapter's opening was actually 2.4 minutes longer than usual, although it was typical in tone.

Most of the time expended during the encounter was filled by the doctor writing in the chart, not conversing with the client. The doctors generally recorded the date of and reason for the visit. For women who had Pap smears, the logistics, such as putting on and taking off gloves or smearing a mucus sample on a slide, followed by a spray of fixant, involved more time than the dialogue between doctor and client. First-time visits that included a breast exam and manual pelvic exam averaged only three minutes. Visits that included a Pap smear in addition to a resupply of a birth control method were on average four minutes in duration.[3] Overall, clients spent only 3 percent of their clinic visit with the doctor. This corroborates Gay's (1980) research in Latin America, which found that time spent with clinicians was often measurable in seconds.

Choice is an important indicator of quality of care, so much so that it stands as a separate element in Bruce's (1989) quality-of-care framework. Family planning specialists consider a wide variety of methods as key to good family planning care. Several phases of clinical and/or acceptability trials have been completed in Haiti: on pills (Pincus et al. 1959), Depo Provera (Tafforeau and Boulos 1986), and Norplant (Klavon and Grub 1990). Because several trials have occurred in Haiti, Haitian women, particularly in urban areas, have been able to choose from an array of contraceptives long before most North American women have had the equivalent choice. The issue of whether an untested or non-FDA–approved method is really a "choice" is questionable when information is generally withheld from clients and clinical research participants.

However choice, in this clinic and most others in Haiti, is typically quantified, measured through inventories of contraceptive stock and commodities. Method choice was, in reality, a statistic reported in a monthly log. Ethnographically observed choice was something quite different. Although many methods were available in the clinic, it did not automatically enhance overall quality of care. Meaningful choice is also bound up in a clinic's ability (and willingness) to offer more than just multiple methods, and depends equally on the clinic's capability of responding to clients' method-specific needs (Simmons and Elias 1994). Although doctors in the family planning center would usually let a woman state her preferred method, they were typically deaf to these requests, and ultimately would choose her method for her. An example of this occurred with Solange, who was thirty-four years old with five children. This was her first visit to the clinic, and she was excited about meeting the doctor. She was smiling when she entered, standing tall, dressed in a clean, crisp white blouse, a mid-calf–length skirt and second-hand high-top tennis shoes. Her smile quickly faded as the doctor began speaking.

DOCTOR: When did you have your period?

CLIENT: I got it Saturday.

D: It's still there?

C: Yes.

D: Do you get it normally, every month?

C: Yes.

D: When it comes, how many days does it usually last?

C: Five, sometimes six days.

D: Have you ever had family planning from another center?

C: No.

D: Go downstairs and they will give you the injectable and return on April 25th. Did they explain the method to you?

C: No.

D: Ok, go downstairs and tell them that.

C: Yes, thank you.

In my sample, the pattern varied little during the course of observation: The doctor generally determined method choice. Some women knew what method they wanted, based on a friend's experience or a conversation with a family planning promoter, but the doctors were quick to override any suggestions or options women would present. Although doctors' choices might often have been medically mandated, there was little, if any, discussion with the patient. A curt *ou pa kapab* (you can't) was the typical response to an expression of choice. Deleting choice of contraceptive from the discussion or failing to elicit information regarding the client's preferred choice served to reinforce doctors' opinions and thus their authority.

If the choice of method is limited for medical reasons, then counseling and providing clear, simple information to clients takes on pronounced importance. The clinic protocol requires women to be menstruating when they receive their packet of pills so that doctors can tell them the exact date to begin taking the cycle of pills. Doctors have told me they do not "trust" women enough to be able to calculate this on their own. However, sending clients away from the clinic without their chosen method of birth control, even if only temporarily, and without an explanation as to why the choice was denied, happened frequently in this setting. New clients were particularly susceptible to this clinic practice. For example, women who were not menstruating (and therefore, due to clinic protocol, could not receive birth control) were often sent from the clinic without their preferred method, typically defeated, and with a stack of condoms in their hand. Although they were told to return when they were menstruating, clients were rarely counseled as to why. Others, who came in for a pregnancy test, fearing pregnancy, were asked to go buy the test, perform it at home, and return with the results (the tests typically cost over US$10). Getting to the pharmacy, finding cash to pay for the test and actually performing a test (from a box with instructions in English or French) was no small feat for a poor resident of Cité Soleil.

The Class Divide: The Socioeconomic Context of Encounters

Power, or lack of it, in an encounter can be viewed in relation to status, authority, and knowledge, all latent dimensions that imbued almost every aspect of doctor-client interaction in this family planning setting. Divides between doctors and clients appeared in different guises—social, economic, and cultural—and stemmed from a general failure of doctors "to criticize the social structural roots of their clients' distress, especially the sources of suffering in class structure" (Waitzkin 1991:22). It was not uncommon for doctors to voice their disdain. At one point, one doctor was deeply frustrated with a client who was confused with his abrupt instructions. When she left the room he looked at me and said, "That woman, she can't read. She's nothing."

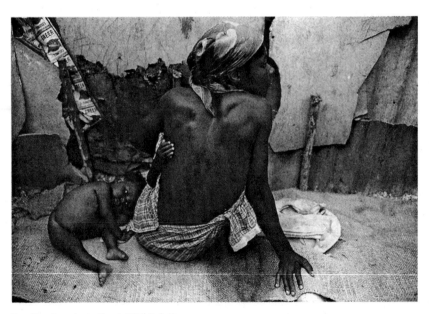

Family planning client, Cité Solcil

Witness the encounter of Simone, who came to the clinic for an injection of Depo-Provera. Carrying her baby on her hip, she entered the examination room with a sad air about her. Frail and worn-looking, an angular face framed her large eyes. Her worn dress was limp, hanging off her bony shoulders and fastened around her waist with a loosely knotted rope. She was twenty-four years old and returned to the clinic following the birth of her child. Her baby, visibly thin with splotches of hair, clung to her skinny arm.

DOCTOR: Have you seen your period?

CLIENT: A little bit of blood came.

D: A small amount?

C: Correct.

D: Are you breastfeeding? You are taking vitamins, right?

C: Well, I don't want to breastfeed anymore.

D: You must breastfeed.

C: But it makes me thin.

D: You're eating, taking vitamins?

C: If you find vitamins. But if you don't have money?

D: But you can't just leave him, when you have a child, especially if he's not yet vaccinated, you have to breastfeed to protect him from diarrhea, to stop the *mikwòb-s* [microbes, germs] from attacking.

C: I'm resigned; I'll take the injectable again.

D: But, but no.

C: I'll take him off the breast, so that I can take that thing.

D: You have to start feeding him, give him lots of liquids, mash up some vegetables and beans and you, eat an egg a day.

C: Where am I going to find these things?

D: How much money do you have?

C: I have five gourdes, I have to pay for the injectable and then I am left with nothing.

D: They'll ask for five gourdes, but you should make a case for only one [gourde]. Go downstairs.

The woman had come, looking for support, wanting to halt her own fast demise brought on by the strains of breastfeeding, hunger, and poverty. Simone's references to her health coincide with Farmer's (1988a) informants' descriptions of *move san* (bad blood), noted here as a chief cause of *lèt gate*, or spoiled milk, syndrome. The syndrome makes it impossible for a nursing mother to provide her infant quality milk and is commonly cited as a motive for early weaning, generally disastrous for infants who have no other nutritive sources. She also tried to contextualize her condition: Her baby who appeared to be dying from malnutrition, her fear of another pregnancy, and worry over her wasting body. She received advice that had little to do with her immediate reality; her circumstances were reduced to a biological event. She worked to bring the conversation back to her reality: "If you find vitamins. But if you don't have money?" and her even more resolute question about the expensive foods recommended— "Where am I going to find these?"

What was particularly poignant about this encounter was that it occurred in the midst of the devastating economic embargo that had, in addition to increasing the poverty of clinic clients, wiped out almost every market vendor in Cité Soleil, a community normally jammed with vendors vying for space, selling everything from herbal medicines to underwear. Many types of food simply were not available—at any price. Almost all women in this study were lucky if they had three meals weekly, not daily. To suggest vegetables, beans, and eggs daily was preposterous even for an elite doctor who at some level also had to be feeling the pinch of the embargo. For a poor woman to "make a case" for paying less than the staff was asking, as the doctor suggested, was equally absurd, since clients, like most Haitian citizens, have no such rights.

Guerta, another client, entered for a consultation. She was experiencing side effects from the injectable. A large and commanding market woman, she looked directly at the doctor, even though he looked at her only at the end of the encounter, when he gave her directions to the nurse's station. During the encounter Guerta almost immediately launched into the subject of persistent bleeding that affected her ability to work in the household: "But the injectable, it gave me bad cramps, and my period flowed and flowed and flowed; it wouldn't stop, I couldn't sit, I couldn't do anything. The other doctor, he gave me pills to take and they did nothing for me." While writing in the chart, the doctor responded, "It [the injectable] can make your period flow more, but it doesn't give you cramps." The client pressed, recounting her experience with the method, although she was ignored. This type of situation occurred repeatedly during observations. Indeed not all clients were entirely diminished in the presence of the physician and some, like Guerta, challenged their power. But clients rarely won in these situations. Repeatedly during encounters, the directed medical discourse would "marginalize the contextual sources of personal distress" (Waitzkin 1991:76).

Typically, clients who did not receive answers from the doctors upstairs would try again downstairs with the nurses, who were less elite than the doctors but still educated and experienced enough to preserve their standing in the social pecking order of the clinic. Though the nurses' responses were often slightly more informative, clients were still met with a measurable degree of contempt. They often left the clinic with unresolved problems, or worse, misunderstandings regarding their health.

Unresolved or misunderstood health conditions were deeply problematic for clients and did little to reinforce a positive clinic experience. The bleeding that Guerta complained of was a recurring theme for many clients during the encounters. Issues around blood flow—either too little or too much—were generally neutralized or ignored by doctors. Several anthropologists working in Haiti have documented the centrality of blood syndromes to concepts of health (Alvarez and Murray 1981; Farmer 1988a). Brodwin (1996:85) notes that the discourse on blood links "powerful emotional states, movements of blood and physical sickness." Heavy bleeding has economic implications as well. A Norplant user, for example, explained her excessive bleeding in terms of too many costs: physical costs that diminished her energy and economic costs from time spent washing her undergarments (which therefore lasted half as long).[4] Repeated washing also cut into valuable market selling time and drained daily finances just to pay for soap. Added to this were serious social costs because her husband, like many other husbands, refused to tolerate the bleeding and left her for another woman.

What was clear from the observed encounters was that authority, medically and technically informed, took precedence over the patients' concerns or reality. Fisher and Todd (1986:8) state it well: "Patients rely on medical practitioners as authorities and medical providers act like authorities." Responding in a technical way, or not at all, was much easier than confronting the real underlying problems women brought to the encounter.

The Cultural Divide: Belittling Beliefs

Though women's economic, physical, and time concerns had little currency for the doctors, concerns related to indigenous cultural beliefs and practices produced even more vast divisions. Repeatedly, a whole array of beliefs and fears related to menstruation, birth, and birth control were dismissed by physicians.

Marie-Marthe entered the consultation room. She was holding a large straw hat and clutching the brim nervously as she spoke to the doctor. She was thirty-two years old and had been a client for over two years. She came to the clinic to resupply her pills but expressed considerable concern about the condition called *move san*.

CLIENT: Well, when I have move san I feel bad and I can't eat.

DOCTOR: You don't have move san, madame.

C: I wasn't sure. I thought maybe the pills were giving me that.

D: It's not the pills. So, is it one packet of pills you'll take this time?

Move san, literally "bad blood," "Begins as a disorder of the blood, but may rapidly spread throughout the body so that head, limbs, eyes, skin, and uterus may all be affected. It most frequently strikes adult women. . . . Although considered pathological, move san is not an uncommon response to emotional upsets. The disorder is seen as requiring treatment, and this is often affected by locally prepared herbal medicines. Untreated or unsuccessfully treated, course and outcome are reported to be dismal" (Farmer 1988a:62).

In another encounter, a client expressed concern with her incessant bleeding caused by *tay ouvè*, literally translated as "open waist." The waist refers to that region of a woman's body that encompasses her reproductive organs and thus her ability to reproduce. Tay ouvè is, according to informants, closely associated with blood loss so severe that it prevents women from being able to bear children, a deeply damaging social stigma among Haitians. Low back stress from carrying heavy loads or excessive work can lead to this condition. Treatments with local "leaf doctors" consist of massages with macerations made of sour oranges followed by wrapping the waist to "close" it. Left untreated, it is said to render women incapable of carrying a child to term. Immediately, the doctor dismissed her self-diagnosis as impossible: "Tay ouvè never makes you bleed like that."

During another encounter, a client made several excuses to avoid a pelvic exam, which the doctor found amusing. "It's an excuse! She's scared a cold wind will enter inside her!" he said to me, smirking. When a Haitian woman gives birth, as this client had done only six weeks earlier, she is "opened up" and takes great care to not *prann frèdi* (take in the cold). In addition to special diets, dress, and the use of herbs for bathing, only certain kinds of activities are warranted until closure is complete. A cloth covers the vagina, and the vaginal region is washed twice daily for forty days. To open oneself up to any other elements is extremely dangerous. And yet the doctor pressed forward to complete the exam, against the client's will.

Generally, cultural concerns, much like clients' socioeconomic plights, were dealt with by interruptions, cutoffs, shifts in tone of voice, or silence. Doctors' negative or mocking reactions were critically important, as they determined whether clients would return for more family planning. When doctors fail to understand women's difficulties, let alone acknowledge their concerns, then the family planning process becomes a deeply disempowering one.

The Reality of Side Effects

Side effects range from merely bothersome to severely debilitating for women everywhere, and typically lead to low rates of contraceptive use. In this realm, the discrepancy between what doctors heard and/or diagnosed and what clients said was striking. According to what the doctors in Cité Soleil recorded in their charts, only 12 percent of the observed women reported side effects. Yet the actual transcriptions revealed that 40 percent had actually reported and enquired about them—often at length, though returning to the clinic for more contraceptives was the main reason recorded for the visit.

Irregular bleeding was the side effect most frequently cited by clients. In this clinic, dismissal of irregular bleeding as a meaningful problem was common and did little to encourage clients to continue method use. Repeatedly, during the collection of data, clients brought their fears, complaints, and concerns to the doctor, only to be met with scorn. The rules of social hierarchy in Haiti dictate that those from the *klas pòv* (lower class) do not normally ask questions of a *moun rich* (rich person). Frequently, clients worked around this by citing examples or mentioning concerns related to methods, though even this tactic yielded little in the way of a response or information.

When Ginette, a twenty-seven-year-old new client with five children, came to the clinic, her anxiety about using Norplant was totally disregarded.

CLIENT: I won't be emptying out? [reference to her blood] I know another woman and she bled for eighteen months straight! Without stopping! She had the five-year method, it emptied her entire body.

DOCTOR: OK, when you return Monday. You will see the nurse downstairs, for Norplant.

C: Please, excuse me?

D: For the five-year method. Go see the nurse downstairs. OK.

Sonite, twenty-two years old, a continuing client using pills, visited the doctor because she hadn't had her period in over four months. She was nervous but determined during the consultation, shifting from side to side, hoping the doctor would offer some resolution to her problem. Her inquiries evoked a stern, paternalistic response.

CLIENT: What I am saying is, if a person doesn't have her period, can you give that person pills to make the period flow?

DOCTOR: Madame. Look, let me ask you a question: What is a period?

C: [laughing nervously] No, I think it can be a real problem, if someone used to get their period and "Plap!" it's gone.

D: OK, let me ask you this, when you were a child and you didn't have a period, did it do anything to you?

C: It didn't do anything because I hadn't yet arrived at the proper age.

D: OK, when you become an old person, fifty or so, you're not twenty anymore, how come you don't have a period?

C: I really think that if you don't have your period it's a problem.

D: There are people who have an operation and remove the entire uterus, you have heard of it? And they don't have a period. Do you see that they die from that? What method do you want, pills again?

In both cases, Ginette and Sonite challenged the doctors' authority and yet doctors were unable to cope when problems could not be technically fixed. Women entered the clinic with serious physical and emotional side effects, but doctors, as evidenced by the cases of Ginette and Sonite, were unable to respond effectively.

Sexually Transmitted Infections and Social Incapacity

Sometimes symptoms perceived as side effects from contraceptive methods actually turned out to be due to sexually transmitted infections (STIs). STIs are common in this population, as they often are where poverty forms the grid of life. Normally, STI screening was not part of the regular service provided to women in the clinic. However, an STI prevalence study was under way during part of the fieldwork period and so the clients in the family planning center benefited from the temporary change in protocol.

Preliminary results of the study showed a high prevalence of many STIs, greater than 60 percent in the community (CDS 1993). In an effort to improve STI case management practices in Haiti, researchers from AIDSCAP, a nongovernmental coalition, CDS, and the University of North Carolina at Chapel Hill (UNC) conducted an evaluation at five of CDS's primary health care centers in Cité Soleil. The study included interviews with health care providers as well as observations of interactions between providers and clients. Clinic and laboratory files were also reviewed as party of the study. "The study revealed that more than 90 percent of the clinicians treated urethral discharge with penicillin or ampicillin, even though tests at the national reference laboratory showed that at least 60 percent of gonococcal strains were resistant to these antibiotics. Treatment of another cause of urethral and vaginal discharge—chlamydia infection—was essentially ignored. Sexual partners of STI patients were seldom referred for treatment, and pregnant women were rarely screened for syphilis" (Behets 2003:1). STIs are a grave health risk for men and women in Cité Soleil (de Zalduondo et al. 1995), and yet the approach to the research in the family planning clinic was perfunctory at best.

During each exam, the language was elliptical. In one instance, the doctor explained the STI study like this, "Tuesday you come here and I will do an exam for you. I'll pass a small stick over your country [vagina] to examine, because they are doing research on the sick and things like that. You understand?"

Sometimes, although not always, the doctor named what he could see—*ti sèvesit*, a "little cervicitis," for example. No information about the disease, its severity, outcome, or treatment options were ever provided. More often he stated, "Madame, you have an infection." The clients always responded "yes," though they appeared confused, frightened, and notably anxious. In follow-up interviews, some clients said they neither understood the origin nor meaning of their STI, which could have serious—even deadly—consequences in the long run. Many of them would grip my arms and plead for an explanation and assistance. Doctors rarely addressed the implications for the other sexual partner, except to say "Don't have sex" or "Have your husband wear a condom."

DOCTOR: What to do. Take tetracycline. If you buy eighty tetracycline you take two in the morning, at noon you take two, in the afternoon you take two— are you listening to what I am telling you?—and in the evening you take two.

CLIENT: In the morning I take two?

D: Like I have written here. Just buy it. The other thing is a cream that you put inside. There are six suppositories in a box. You buy it in the pharmacy. At *Pharmacie Vallière* you can find it.

C: What's it called?

D: You get it wet and then you put it inside. If you have your period don't use it. And when you put it in, don't have any sexual relations, no sex.

C: Yes, if I have, wait until my period? Before I . . .?

D: You'll look to see how many times to take it.

Similar in content to countless other encounters, the doctor failed to identify the STI (this client had candida and gonorrhoea), and he did not take the time needed to explain the treatment effectively. The doctor also assumed that the woman could read instructions, forgetting that most of his clients are illiterate. Even more disturbing, filling the prescription was nearly impossible. The cost of a single Tetracycline prescription—approximately US$30—at the time was very high, especially when food was such a priority.

The doctors' insistence on not having sex (or telling women to demand condom use of their partners, as they frequently did) assumed that women exercise significant control within the reproductive and sexual realms of their lives. STIs, like problematic side effects, function as symbols of social incapacity, bringing to the foreground how disease undermines poor women on so many fronts. Marie Ange clarified this, describing what is a "right" for women: "Oh sure, you've got the right to ask them to put on a condom, and when they don't want to, then you don't want to. It's not a matter of insisting because they beat you; this is the progress that women have made. They beat you, they sleep with you, they *mawon* you [literally 'maroon,' to flee into hiding], and you are left pregnant."

Even more telling were the comments the doctor made after the patient left the room. I asked:

CATHERINE MATERNOWSKA: Do you always choose tetracycline for gonorrhoea?

DOCTOR: Not always, because there are lots of choices for STIs. It depends on their economic means. Tetracycline is the best buy. You give it as necessary, between 80 and 120 pills per treatment.

CM: Is that the normal dose, eight pills a day for ten days or more? Are there side effects?

D: Well you can have side effects but you have them eat when they take it, out of necessity. Or you can give them Canistotine [unclear] 250 mg a one-time shot and you're finished. But it costs $45 a box plus the syringe. It's all a choice.

It was a choice in the doctor's mind, but for poor clients there is very little, if any, choice at all. Choice in Cité Soleil for a woman with a reproductive or sexually related infection is infinitely more complicated than the way doctors see it. "No matter how convenient family planning or reproductive health services are, if women can't afford them, they will not have a significant impact" (Richey 1999a:206). Emilienne reminded me of how the poor cope with their severely limited financial options. Twenty-six years old, with two children and no steady partner, she visited the clinic for what she thought might be an infection. She looked frightened, twisting a pink plastic shopping sack around her hands as she spoke to me. "Are you a doctor?" she asked, her eyebrows tightly knit. She showed me how a poor household tries to manage sickness: "I have no money, and I am sick. That's why I am selling these." Inside the dirty bag were her four year-old daughter's little shoes. "They're used," she said, looking down.

Family Planning as an Institution: Social Context and the Staff

Issues of power, authority, and class imbue every aspect of the client-provider interaction. These issues, however, were not contained within the consultation rooms—they also wedged themselves between and among the staff, recreating Haiti's pervasive social hierarchy and creating an institutional context that was deeply divisive.

Nowhere was this clearer than during staff meetings—the only time when all staff members convened in the same room at the same time. The doctor who directed the clinic was dressed in a shirt and tie, with pressed slacks and freshly polished shoes. When he formerly worked as a clinician he would often joke with the clients and engage in their lives. Frequently he would go out of his way to help someone in need. He was a dòk (doctor) that everyone loved. As the son of two farmers, he was one of the lucky (and few) brilliant students who actually made it into Haiti's state-managed medical school without ties to the upper classes. Years of working at this clinic and dealing with the rigorous demands of international agencies had slowly transformed this man from a humble, client-devoted doctor to a hard, urban bureaucrat who directed the clinic.

There were no tables in the room, just the doctor's desk pushed into a corner. The staff sat on brown folding chairs, formed in a circle. Everyone was at attention and completely silent, staring ahead. A large nurse wiped sweat dripping from her forehead with a handkerchief. The clinic director began the meeting: "[Contraceptive] prevalence has dropped to 5 percent. We need to work harder. I measure someone's success by the number of clients they bring in." Everyone maintained his or her stoic positions. No one responded to his comment. He paused, then folded his arms and shifted his body.

His gaze moved to the promoters, responsible for community recruitment but also the most poorly paid and overworked of all the clinic staff. Suddenly he barked, "What's happening?" A daring promoter spoke out, "Well, it seems our supervisors act more aristocratic than us—they don't even say hello." Referring to an auxiliary nurse who served as the promoters' supervisor, the promoter continued: "If she's going to be our supervisor, then she should be going out with us every day. She should be writing a report and we should be allowed to give a report, too." The supervisor remained silent and looked almost catatonic, staring ahead at the wall, her lips tightly pursed, her ankles tightly crossed. The promoters merely wanted support—and acknowledgment—for their work. And yet they were blamed for their inabilities to recruit clients and shunned by virtue of their status as poor women from the community.

The discussion quickly became heated. All of the promoters jumped to speak, all of them decidedly angry. Chaos ensued, complete with yelling and gesturing; one nurse was clapping her hands above her head, trying to bring order, and the Norplant nurse was shrieking in a high-pitched voice, "Over 45 percent of the clients come in on their own," further implying that the promoters had little to do with client activity. The two staff doctors sat together, slightly apart from the rest of the group, both slouched with their chins in their hands, completely silent and disengaged, showing no facial expression in the midst of this chaos. Never once did anyone pause to assess what might be wrong *inside* the clinic and how inappropriate, or simply insufficient, services might be for poor clients.

What was most evident during this meeting and several others that followed was how the professional rank and associated class of the staff served to distance the promoters at every level, ensuring poor staff communication and ultimately distrust. Doctors provided strictly technical skills—those endowed by their prestigious medical degrees. Their behavior was one of clear disassociation with the rest of the clinic staff. In fact, never during the entire period of observation did a doctor actually consult with a nurse about a client's case. The nurses, in turn, spoke in negative terms about auxiliaries, because auxiliaries lacked the professional training that nurses had. Auxiliaries, in separate interviews, indicated that the family planning promoters lacked education. In fact, promoters were largely uneducated and had been trained through informal educational structures. They possessed only a certificate with a gold paper emblem and script writing, given to them following a course with a local nongovernmental organization. All of the promoters proudly displayed their certificates on the walls of their humble homes, since this was often the only recognition they ever received.

The doctors and nurses represent the dominant class: the wealthy, French-speaking cosmopolitan minority. The auxiliary nurse, without any real power, falls somewhere in between, in Haiti's small, forgotten, and increasingly poor middle class. The promoters represent the poor, black, and (in this case) barely literate masses. The clients, unfortunately, fall between the cracks of these "two worlds." They become inconsequential—targets, numbers, and ultimately percentages reflected in monthly service reports demanded by international agencies. Clients are objectified and treatment depersonalized, devoid of respect or dignity. But the promoters and the clients (and potential clients) are all poor women who share, by history and birth, a common misery in this community.

Key here is that the clinic *depends* on promoters and their recruits, these deeply disdained representatives of the masses. The family planning center is a microcosm of a much larger codependency that runs deep through Haitian society. Although there is an ongoing international controversy around the issue of race in the social sciences, and more recently in public health debates, I deliberately do not address it in this analysis. In Haiti, issues of both color and class have been prominent forces, historically and in the present. This study, however, is driven by a class analysis because participants, especially the poor women, always spoke of class distinctions, typically referring to the elite as educated and powerful. Inside the clinic too, the pronounced pecking order among the staff, based on class, status, and education, mirrors Haitian society. Fatton calls this divide the "two worlds" of Haiti. He continues (Fatton 2002:52–53), "The second world is defined in relation to the dominant class; it is dependent on it and subject to it. At the same time, the first world's wealth and status derive from its control and taxation of the poor majority. First and second worlds are thus bound together in unequal but interdependent relationships that have generated an enormous gap between the haves and the have-nots."

When asked about perspectives on population growth and Haitian society, the staff appeared to be informed. In interviews they saw the problem of low family planning use as having social and economic roots. "It's simple," said a nurse, "when the economy falls, then fertility rises." A doctor lamented, "It's a global problem; our economic structure has never been in place, and in fact we are worse off now than we were ten years ago. High unemployment and a lack of education serve to support big families, and I predict the hunger and the babies will continue for many years to come." And yet, the understanding of macro forces was distinctly removed from the micro situation in the clinic—or the community—and their analyses did not appear to inform their treatment or discussion of clients. Indeed their analyses confirmed an enormous gap between insight and practice.

Although both the nurses acknowledged the difficult life the poor lead and made connections to a lack of education for the largely illiterate population, their comments were shrouded with righteous judgments. They elaborated negatively on sexual strategies women employ to survive. One nurse commented that she felt it was "immoral" for women to have children by several different fathers, even though this was the norm among clients. Another nurse commented: "There's a tendency to be a (loose woman, prostitute) . . . to look for a man so as to give him a child . . . They shouldn't be prostitutes, they should find another way."

The nurse in charge of counseling saw women as "very empowered" in Haiti, but when I asked about the status of women in Cité Soleil, the conversation shifted to the nurse's own class. In the midst of her analysis she subconsciously shifted into French, rather than Creole, the language in which I was interviewing. "Of course women are equal to men, women in Haiti have evolved to an equal level with men, they work outside of the home, and they can even say to their husbands, 'I only want two children'—like me, I decided." The statistics that I had collected painted a decidedly different picture. Unable and unwilling to analyze the needs of her patients, the nurse refused to address the social, economic, or political conditions of the poor. She effectively ensured her distance by feigning ignorance or practicing denial. Even when I probed and described to her the hand-to-mouth economy that I had witnessed, along with women's poor status in the household, she dismissed my observations with a wave of her hand. Smiling at me, and in a joking and somewhat condescending manner, she said, "*Ah Kati, ou se yon moun fou—fou pou pòv yo.*" She called me "crazy for the poor," conveniently acknowledging that my "craziness" and any questions associated with it were my problem, not hers.

Attitudes toward the clients, particularly those of the nurses and auxiliaries, were often no different than those of the doctors. Gossip in the nursing station often slid into derisive comments about certain clients. Moral judgments were common in the clinic. When a poor, sick woman arrived in the nursing station, the nurse yelled out to me, "Look at this *ti malerèz* (poor woman), six children! Ohhh! They never stop! Madame, why do you keep having children?" Morality—another form of authority—often turned to blaming, such as with Justine, who wanted pills but could not use them because of varicose veins, a contraindication to pill use. The nurse was quick to pipe in, "It's because you have five children that you have those veins." Once a nurse looked at me as a client was leaving and pinched her nose in disgust.

Moral judgments did little to improve the clinic experience, yet filling clients with shame seemed almost commonplace and habitual. Following an encounter, which was replete with derogatory remarks, a young couple (the only couple that I had ever seen in the clinic) returned downstairs to the nursing station for a new supply of pills. One of the nurses called out to me, "Look at these two, they're babies! What? Family planning for little children! Oh! They shouldn't be having relations!"

The auxiliary nurses in the clinic—who are professionals wedged considerably below the status of a nurse in Haiti, and considerably above that of a family planning promoter—declined to be interviewed for the study. On observation they appeared bossy with the clients, and their rapport with the promoters, whom they managed, was strained. I suggested to the doctor that the auxiliary nurses join the promoters during house-to-house visits. Once they did, their rapport improved remarkably. According to one promoter, the auxiliary who had the field experience was shocked by the intensity and difficulty of the work *nan mitan mizè* (in the midst of poverty).

The family planning promoters, also part of the center's staff, were a team of nine women, all living in Cité Soleil. Without their community-based recruitment and regular client follow-up, the family planning program would have ceased to exist. The promoters' work was grueling, within harsh physical conditions of hot sun or flooding, depending on the season, and a very densely packed population. Promoters were well aware of their own status, nearly, if not equally, as low as that of the poor women who entered the clinic. Promoters were frequently mistreated by other staff, looked down upon, and rarely given the respect they deserved for their difficult work.

Naturally, the work of the promoters, deep inside the community, linked them to the realm of the social, economic, and political realities of life in Cité Soleil. They found this both difficult and disturbing, particularly since hunger and political repression—not family planning—were foremost in people's minds. Like other clinic staff, their explanations of high fertility and low contraceptive use were based on political and economic reality, but with a more grounded sense of urgency: "People are multiplying and we can go on forever giving them education and telling them they'll suffer less, but they'll still have more [children]. It's the political crisis that has degenerated our lives. No money, no food—poor women are obliged to offer their bodies and they are dying with AIDS."

Unfortunately, even the family planning promoters, impoverished women themselves, were observed adopting judgmental attitudes toward noncompliant clients, possibly to defend their just slightly higher status in the social hierarchy. Sometimes during group counseling sessions the promoters would become haughty, deriding clients for not understanding menstruation, for example. This behavior was considerably more pronounced when they worked inside the clinic, especially when other clinic staff were listening. Still, the promoters' extremely difficult work conditions, very low pay, and physical closeness to the clients made them the most understanding and compassionate workers on the staff.

Quality of Care Revisited

Family planning programs, largely the responsibility of the medical profession, tend to approach fertility reduction as a straightforward issue of compliance with medical recommendation. Often, medical professionals (and likewise international health and development experts who design these interventions) assign blame to women who "fail" to comply with doctors' orders. The quality-of-care framework was purported to reframe the focus from blaming the client to the program, to ensure that services were good enough to attract and satisfy clients. In this way, the framework—now the gold standard of reproductive health discourse—was promoted as a way to provide services that truly addressed women's reproductive needs.

In a critical review of clinic activities in Tanzania, Richey (1999a:181) makes a cogent point: "[The quality-of-care] framework still situates family planning as viewed from a demographically-driven, 'negative' perspective. It is meant to combat the population 'problem' by enabling women to have fewer children. The emphasis on quality is simply a motivator for these women on whom the responsibility rests for solving the 'problem.' The realm for understanding quality of care is assumed to be at the individual level, not at the larger social, economic, or political levels."

When critically analyzed, medical encounters and the institutional dynamics that surround them show how contraceptive behavior is influenced by myriad forces—social, economic, cultural, and ultimately political. Clients' reproductive decision making was curtailed or, worse, negated as they proceeded through the health care system. While population agencies embrace the quality-of-care framework, "in the absence of a functioning health care system, it is difficult, if not impossible, to have a decent family planning program with adequate screening and follow-up" (Hartmann 1995:136). Add to this reality political and economic instability, and women's reproductive options were diluted even further. So-called quality of care, in the Haitian context, serves primarily to distract the medical and development community from more pressing issues around reproductive rights. This distraction amounts to yet another form of structural violence (Doyal 1995; Farmer 2002; Scheper-Hughes 1992).

And yet USAID and its collaborating agencies press forward with the quality-of-care framework. In theory, the framework provides a provocative platform from which to analyze programs, as I have here. But, as both Richey and Hartmann argue, in practice a realistic look at "quality" is problematic in a country where the infrastructure barely merits the name. In January 2002, a conference directed specifically at the six elements of the framework and "putting clients first" was held at a popular beach resort outside the capital. The objectives of the meeting were to examine specific elements of quality service and "on the eve of the new 5-year bilateral program to make recommendations for improved RH [reproductive health] services for Haitian women and families" (JHPIEGO 2000:1). The most noteworthy item on the agenda, under the entry "interaction between client and provider," were the questions: "What is the reality of the client-provider interaction? How far is the reality from the ideal?"

A review of the elements of the quality-of-care framework in the Cité Soleil clinic shows just how far reality can be from an ideal, especially in the context of poverty.

- *Choice of methods* is limited by a person's means or by the doctor who dictates to patients what method they will use.
- *Information given to clients* is provided primarily by the family-planning promoters, who are ill-equipped to handle many biomedical concerns, so the majority of women's questions go unanswered. In the rare cases where doctors do inform, client concerns are ignored.

- *Technical competence*, measured by "meticulous asepsis required to provide clinical methods," in the face of no electricity or running water, was nothing short of absurd.
- *Interpersonal relations* between staff and clients were strained at best, as were relations among all levels of clinic personnel.
- *Mechanisms to encourage continuity* were absent, since family planning was not placed within a broader context of reproductive and sexual health (Hardon and Hayes 1997).
- *The appropriate constellation of services* was doomed from the start, since preexisting health needs were simply never addressed.

In resource-deficient settings, where high fertility is more an effect of—rather than a cause of—poverty, the quality-of-care framework may be theoretically useful but practically inappropriate. By vigorously promoting "quality" in the Haitian context, international agencies are doing what "first-world" privileged Haitians do—distancing themselves from the reality just outside the clinic doors. Improving one element, or even all six, will not fix Haiti's population problem. There are too many factors—related to class and political economy—that have everything to do with why women and men can't "control" their own reproduction. The family planning center in Cité Soleil, as seen through the medical encounters that occur there, replicates the structures that condemn the poor, wherever they go. Worse, even if this clinic did presumably "improve" one or all of the quality-of-care elements in some clinically distilled way, then managers, program planners, and even policy makers would, as is often the case in Haiti, absolve themselves as part of the problem. In the end, this would conveniently push the onus back onto the shoulders of the "noncompliant" poor or the hard-working clinic staff.

What's Making People Sick?

Having found one of the seemingly rare men who both supported family planning and his wife's desire to use it, I asked for his analysis of why so few people used family planning in Cité Soleil. Olike was a forty-two-year-old man who had resided in Cité Soleil since 1985. With the equivalent of a junior high education, Olike was formerly employed in a factory for what was then a wage of US$3 a day but he lost his job when the company closed. When we talked, he sat outside his meager shack wearing maroon-colored polyester trousers and a silky seventies disco shirt. His wide and calloused feet balanced him as he leaned back in the frame of a chair that had only six dirty ropes woven in the seat area. He had attended the clinic with his wife on two separate visits, which informed his analysis. His arms were crossed and occasionally he gestured with a pointed finger. He began,

> It all depends on who organizes the family planning services, because they are poorly organized. First, it's clear that the few people who actually

use the services don't benefit from them. Someone's always talking about what sickness they have from planning, so it's not surprising that no one goes. If *planin* were a positive experience, then one would encourage the other to go. You understand how our country works. We honor what works, and if the services were good, we would embrace the organization. Instead, people run from that place.

Second, we all know that the center has money in it, but to what end? For its own purposes. You know this is a country where we have no economy, a plight we don't deserve. That [family planning] organization has a huge base of money and they should be able to offer good services.

Third, it seems to me that *planin* has little to do with satisfying people's real needs. They [the doctors] don't probe or ask questions; they just see if you deserve a prescription and then give it to you, never inquiring about everything that's really making you sick. There is no concern for those who are suffering. People who go to the doctor have problems. What's important is not to judge a person for not having money, but to appreciate the person—really, *to understand their life* (author's emphasis).

Olike's pointed criticisms further confirmed what this study has assumed all along: that looking at family planning programs in the context of people's lives is critical. Without this sort of analysis reproductive health needs will likely go unaddressed, along with all the other things "making" people sick.

This chapter has shown how low contraceptive use is far more than just a compliance or "quality-of-care" issue. Attempts to improve this clinic have centered almost exclusively on the technology and its most efficient delivery. But more flipcharts, speculate, or family planning promoters will do little to change the complex and deeply embedded structural issues that give shape to people's contraception-related experiences. The small percentage of women who withstand household pressures and decide to use family planning are not rewarded for their perseverance. The power that providers claim in the encounter reminds clients that they are unworthy, even "animals," a description used to castigate one client who wanted to discontinue her method of birth control. Because doctors' directive power is so forceful, clients are systematically denied information they need to participate actively in their reproductive health. If anything, these encounters serve to remind poor Haitian women of their marginalization. When they reach home, the inequity in gender relations inevitably reinforces the extent to which Haitian women are disenfranchised.

Applying a political economy framework to assess traditional family planning issues helps analyze program impacts, situating caregivers and receivers in their larger social, political, and economic contexts. When the program is viewed as a political arena, it becomes clear that relations of power in the clinic shape the manner in which health care is both provided and perceived. One of the great claims of family planning is that it empowers women and men to make choices and control their own fertility. In Cité Soleil, the quality of the program and its relationship with the community did little to support that claim. Rather than empowering clients to gain control of their reproductive lives, this program effectively prohibited the poor from broadening their base of power or gaining social support for their decision to use contraceptives.

Olike's lament that the clinic "ha[d] little to do with satisfying people's real needs" was in fact a widespread sentiment in Cité Soleil. From the perspective of the poor, the family planning center embodied all that was wrong with the way public health was delivered, and its presence in the community, as we will see, did not go uncontested.

5

A Community Consumed

Fire, Politics, and Health Care

> Health is a profoundly political issue, but it is often in the interests of those who control health policy to perpetuate the illusion that health is immune to political considerations.
>
> —Lynn Morgan, "'Political Will' and Community
> Participation in Costa Rican Primary Health Care"

Transistor radios are prized possessions in Haiti. For the majority of Haitians who cannot read or write, radios educate. When the coup d'état of 1991 erupted, radio announcers were among the first attacked. The illegal de facto regime immediately seized control of the airwaves (America's Watch Committee [US] and National Coalition for Haitian Refugees 1993). After that, listening to the news on the radio—poor Haitians' single connection to the outside world—was a crime punishable by beatings and even death.

Music, however, was permissible. For months, news was transmitted into the country through the Dominican Republic. Progressive radio broadcasters working from the border would transmit reports of events, and often political messages, encoded in the lyrics of songs. For at least a year following the coup, on a fairly regular basis at 7:30 a.m. on Tropique FM residents of Cité Soleil would move and smile—a wry smile—to *We We*, a jazzy African song by Angélique Kidjo from Benin. The lyrics, translated, go like this:

Fire burns in our hearts, fire burns in our houses.
They say it's for reasons of the state.
They say it's in the name of justice.
Today torturers are everywhere: Tomorrow who will judge them?
Fire burns in our hearts, fire burns in our houses.

To discern the meaning of this song, particularly for residents of Cité Soleil, is to understand how they came to be consumed by fire, politics, and health care.

Urban Planning, Haitian-Style

Housing is the most visible dimension of poverty in Cité Soleil, even though the community was explicitly created to provide "improved" housing conditions for the growing urban poor. In September 1951, the Haitian government under President Magloire passed a law to develop an administrative office for the creation of "worker cities" (Maingrette 1995). Cité Simone (originally named in honor of Madame Simone Duvalier, the wife of Papa Doc) was one of the communities slated for construction in the late 1950s, under the newly formed Duvalier government.

The construction of Cité Simone, for an estimated population of 5,000 workers, was the idea of several powerful Haitian-Arab merchants. These merchants had long eyed La Saline, a neighboring slum, just across from the waterfront, as a prime site for a vast commercial plaza. The fact that thousands of rural peasants lived in La Saline posed some problems: Their houses were built on property with potentially high commercial value. Under the Papa Doc government, the minister of health, also of Haitian-Arab descent, began one of the capital's first urban housing projects, constructing dwellings in what is now Cité Soleil. He rallied support within the Haitian-Arab community, "people he did business with," says Father Arthur Volel, a Salesian priest who worked in both La Saline and Cité Simone. The goal was to move the *mas pèp la* (popular masses) from one slum to another so that the development of La Saline could serve the economic interests of the elite.

The homes constructed for Cité Simone's first inhabitants were of good quality, according to older residents, complete with functioning latrines. Even so, people living in La Saline generally chose not to uproot, because moving to Cité Simone was an isolating prospect (La Saline was located near a road with access to areas where the poor were employed). A former resident recalls, "There was no transportation in those days; the poor walked everywhere." Unable to persuade the residents of La Saline to move, the state eventually sold the Cité Simone houses mostly to rural peasants staking a life in Port-au-Prince. Father Volel, then a young priest sent by his order to live in this new community, recalled with disdain, "They were nice little houses, but then the people started disturbing things. They built additions on their houses and then they built more houses, even in the narrow alleys." Nearly a decade later, the population of Cité Simone had doubled.

Rural-to-urban migration continued, and so too did the growth of La Saline. In December 1967, the first of several mysterious fires was set in La Saline, to permanently "solve" the problem. A second and then a third fire, on the December 17, destroyed everything in the La Saline slum. "Their little straw houses were demolished within minutes," says Volel. The urban planning project was complete.

The now-wrinkled priest laughed nervously and asked me to turn off my tape recorder in order to tell me that these fires, and others, were all state-sponsored events, headed by the chief of one of the most infamous *tonton makout-s* (armed militia), Madame Max Adolphe. Madame Max, as she was called, was then the warden of Fort Dimanche, a notorious Duvalier prison where "thousands of the Duvaliers' enemies had languished, starved, and died, if they were not simply tortured and executed" (Wilentz 1989:119). Fort Dimanche, not coincidently, stands on the salt flats opposite La Saline. Volel, quick to defend Madame Max, indicated that she offered free transportation into Cité Simone for the homeless victims.

The needs of this community, particularly in terms of public health, were extensive. In response, the Haitian Arab Center was incorporated in 1974 as a nongovernmental organization with its offices in Cité Simone. The former minister of health who helped create the original housing community managed it. In a bulletin praising the efforts of the Haitian government, he referred to Cité Simone as "a large and magnificent piece of land" (Maingrette 1995:8), though the residents there have always thought differently. The former minister's training in medicine and public health was immediately applied. So, too, was the assistance of his sons, several of whom had become physicians or pharmacists who had received public health training in the United States. Later, the Haitian Arab Center expanded to become the Medical Social Complex of Cité Simone, which worked closely with the Michèle B. Duvalier Foundation and eventually evolved into what is now called CDS, the French acronym for the Centres pour le Développement et la Santé (Centers for Health and Development).

The change of name from Cité Simone to Cité Soleil came with the political change that ousted the Duvalier family from power in 1986 (in a relatively non-violent coup). The new name, Cité Soleil, was a popular decision that referred to Radyo Soley, the progressive Catholic radio station, among the first in the country to beam news to the poor residents in Haitian Creole rather than French.

"We're Perishing": Water, Hunger, and the Grid of Poverty

At the turn of the millennium, the public health needs of Cité Soleil remain extensive. Overcrowding and a lack of basic infrastructure mark all of the neighborhoods in Cité Soleil. "*Ah . . . n ap peri*" (Ah . . . we're perishing), exclaimed Denise, a nineteen-year-old mother of one child who lived in one of the community's most deprived neighborhoods. She looked up and said something I had heard hundreds of times before, "*M pa gen kòb*" (I have no money).

Statistically and practically speaking, Denise was correct. People inside Cité Soleil are nearly perishing. At the time of data collection, unemployment in Cité Soleil peaked at 80 percent, and the cost of living doubled following the coup d'état of 1991.[1] Her statement reflects the difficulty residents faced as they struggled to manage the delicate balance of inputs (usually cash) and outputs (usually marketed and nonmarketed goods and services) required to maintain a household and, by extension, a community. In this hand-to-mouth economy, the most pressing needs for daily survival, apart from housing, focused on the basics of finding food and water. During times of crisis, these basic needs were common to almost all residents, making survival a community effort.

Over 80 percent of Cité Soleil is situated on swampy, marshy land. There are several large canals that resemble moats and traverse many of the neighborhoods. The water is black, fetid, and highly polluted, since these canals are the sites of both animal and human defecation and used as general garbage dumps in which pigs wander. For lack of other sources, people sometimes bathe in this water. Other areas of Cité Soleil border the Bay of La Gonave, and are generally the poorest and most waterlogged neighborhoods, where malaria is endemic. Public water facilities are very limited. Only seven of fifty-two people interviewed had access to water spigots inside Cité Soleil, and usually they were people in good graces with the nuns.[2] The main method of obtaining water was to buy it from one of several hundred water sellers who transported it daily from surrounding neighborhoods in buckets on their heads. The purchase of water was costly. For example, laundry, ideally done on a weekly basis, required the purchase of six buckets at Hg 2/bucket (US$0.14), the equivalent of one fairly prosperous day of labor for a market woman. During the embargo things got worse, when the population with access to potable water in Port-au-Prince declined from 52 percent in 1990 to 35 percent in 1994 (Farmer and Smith Fawzi 2002).

When asked about food and meals, women invariably kicked the recho (the handmade three-legged container that during prosperous times held burning charcoal as the foundation of a cooked meal). Hands on their hips, many women angrily exclaimed, "*M pa menm monte chodyè*" (I don't even use my cooking pot). Indeed during my fieldwork, cooking a meal was a huge event and soon became a communally shared event.

In order to cook a meal, cash had to be secured to buy essential ingredients. To do this, Haitians have, over the decades, devised various means of short-term financial survival, since banks in Haiti generally do not serve the country's majority poor. One of the most popular schemes for pooling resources was the traditional *sòl*, a tried-and-tested form of Haitian reciprocal group lending. Members of a sòl, usually around ten or so, give approximately US$1 to a common pot on a given day of the week. One person each week receives the entire group's investment, bringing a relatively large cash influx to that member. The same process begins in the next week, and another person from the group is the recipient of the cash. Nearly all households were surviving on sòl, since enormous amounts of energy—physical energy that people simply did not have—had to be expended to bring in US$1 or less a day to a household. Of women interviewed, 71 percent were making less than one dollar per day. In 1993, less than one dollar could not stave off family hunger in Cité Soleil. None of the men were employed.

To understand the actual meaning of the "cost of living" in the community, I joined experienced shoppers in the market, giving them Hg75 (approximately US$5.25) to spend, and recording their purchases. Rosie was able to purchase the following for her household of nine members (three adults and six children): a small basket of twelve plantains, four onions, four tomatoes, three cups of cornmeal, four bouillon seasoning cubes, and a cup of sugar. This did not include the purchase of charcoal or matches, both required to cook the food. By her estimates, market prices had quadrupled since the coup.

When prepared, meals were commonly divided not only within a household but also among households comprising close kin and extended kin and the usual several "charity" cases, most often hungry neighbors. Although it was rare actually to witness the preparation of a hot meal during the embargo, it was an event when it occurred. I spent one morning talking to Yolette while she prepared a meal. When I asked what she was making, she told me: *fokseli*, a national dish in times of poverty, made with cooked milled corn served with a bean sauce, when money permits. We sat in a narrow corridor and leaned against a cement block wall. It was extremely hot inside the "kitchen," with the boiling pot on the fire and the sun pounding down on us. When the wind blew, the fumes stung our eyes. With the household's single knife, she deftly peeled the skin from the onion, careful to discard only the very driest layer. Her upbeat manner was palpable. She admitted to me that she was feeling particularly useful that day as a mother and provider in her role as cook. "At least today, we will eat," she said managing a smile. When the food was ready, she used pieces of torn corrugated cardboard as pot holders and moved the heavy metal pot to the floor.

Once the food cooled some, she began to serve it, squatting before the pot. Dipping a small plastic bowl into the large pot, she measured the mush very carefully into twelve other small plastic bowls and two larger plates (for the men). When this meticulous process was finished, she looked at me and eloquently summed up the process with a proverb: *manje kwit pa gen mèt* (cooked food belongs to no one). Smith (2001) calls these proverbs that pepper the Creole language "collective mantras" of daily conversation, and they are almost always based on sharing. In reality, though, many families in the community survived on dry crackers and sugar-cane water, both of which had the deceiving effect of "filling" the consumer's stomach. Malnutrition was endemic; people were often folded over in pain from gastric ulcers, a direct effect of hunger.

During times of crisis Haitians call on one another—*yon ede lòt* (one helping another). Although many associate this interdependence and cooperation with rural Haiti (Smith 2001), it was very common in Cité Soleil. Community responses to hunger included the creation of survival organizations, called *oganizasyon popilè* (popular organizations), such as communal kitchens and community credit groups to help the poor secure loans. All of these organizations operated clandestinely out of fear stemming from political instability and repression (cf. Paley 2001). The groups that I knew in Cité Soleil were funded through international solidarity organizations, nonprofit organizations, or by a connection to a *blan* (foreigner), usually an American or French person with some compassion and a little cash. The size of these popular organizations, many of them run by women, could be as small as ten and as large as one hundred. Usually one member's house was designated as a meeting place. During repressive times larger groups were divided into smaller groups to keep the security risk low. Groups would come together in what became known as a *tet ansanm* (cooperative team) to reflect on the lack of social justice in Cité Soleil and the country at large. These organizations gave meaning to people's struggle to survive and helped political activists and advocates feel cohesively joined in their own form of *demokrasi*, in spite of all the repression.

Often I would visit with the members of one very active community association made up of several dozen poor women, all residents of Port-au-Prince slums. As members, they provided mutual solidarity and support at a time when their greatest feat was keeping their children alive. They were determined to organize for better lives. Elita, president and spokesperson of the organization said this: "Right now we have educational projects. One of us knows how to sew, and she is teaching the others, but she needs money for cloth and needles and thread. Another woman is good at baking bread and pastries, but she doesn't have money to buy the materials she needs. Also, we have a nurse with us. And we have a literacy project. We are rich in knowledge but short on tools. We want one day to build a small house, a place for our group to meet."

And yet organizing—even to stave off hunger—was a complicated process. All of the structural forces in Haiti that bombard the poor, and especially poor women, were constantly present. If nothing else, these meetings helped reinforce the concept of "one helping another": Françoise (a young member of Elita's organization) wanted me to understand how they grappled with poverty in both practical and analytical terms: "When our group meets, we really put our heads together. We try to figure out why some are selling more than others, to learn so we can sell better. And we try to help one another. Some women come to our meetings and cry; they tell us their husbands are giving them problems. We say, " 'Women weren't made to cry because of men. If he gives you problems, give him problems right back!' "

Map Kalkile (I'm Calculating): The Economics of Health Care

As individuals and as members of survival organizations, residents of Cité Soleil always *kalkile*. Kalkile has several meanings in Creole—to think (over), reflect and consider, as well as to calculate, compute, or estimate. All of these meanings have much to do with community survival. Often, residents would assume the kalkile position—sitting quietly, backs very straight, looking directly ahead.

Calling out to greet a friend, *Ki jan ou ye?* (How are you doing?), the response would frequently be: *Ah, map kalkile* (Ah, I am calculating). Indeed, survival in the midst of poverty is a very precisely calculated effort, right down to the last penny. Against the grim possibilities of actually finding work, food, or water, health remains a constant preoccupation for residents in Cité Soleil. It is in this domain that calculations are most critical.

"Can you tell me three sicknesses that are likely to affect adults in this community?" I asked. Marie Dedette, twenty-two years old and a mother of two children, responded: "There aren't three illnesses, there are only two: *maladi grangou* (hunger sickness) and *maladi seksyèl* (sexually transmitted infections)." The absence of health in Cité Soleil is obvious: big-bellied children and fever-ridden adults are a common sight. There are also, increasingly, more latent diseases. HIV infection prevalence is said to be as high as 10.5 percent among healthy women receiving prenatal care in this community (Boulos et al. 1990). Untreated sexually transmitted infections (STIs) result in systemic afflictions that weaken immune systems, leaving the already vulnerable even more so (Brutus 1989). Other commonly diagnosed illnesses include arthritis and hernias from carrying heavy loads, malaria from stagnant water pools, and tuberculosis and other airborne viruses from cramped living quarters. Bernard et al. (1993), in his study of Cité Soleil, listed colds, malaria, "fever," diarrhea, hypertension, typhoid, and tuberculosis as the most commonly cited diseases among respondents (cf. Lerebours and Canez 1992).[3]

When I asked Josette the same question about the three main sicknesses in the community, she distilled her answer even further: *maladi peyi a* (the country's sickness). Elaborating, she talked about the simple absence of opportunity. "Just look around you," she said, gesturing to her children naked and covered with flies. Although this response did not fit into standard public health survey rhetoric, it resolutely reflected the nature of structural imbalances and the unhealthy impact these imbalances impose on people's lives and bodies in this community.

Reports detailing the work of CDS in Cité Soleil claim that the poor had good access to health care in this community. As a nation, Haiti has only one physician for every 7,140 people (UNDP 1994). In Cité Soleil, the statistics are impressively better, with at least one physician to every 2,195 people—a standard three times as high as the national average. The infrastructure and staffing were impressive: five health centers (this included the family planning center), a hospital, eighty-two physicians (many of them specialists), four medical clinics, and seven community pharmacies. Doctors, nurses, auxiliaries, and community health agents associated with these medical facilities employed multiple strategies, from clinic-based appointments to community-based home visits with outreach and follow-up to track the health status of entire households. If a community resident wanted to use CDS services, the entire family was required to register to ensure full family coverage. A *carte de famille* (family card) was supplied and listed the household address, along with the names and ages of each household member. Some of the clinics had additional cards that mothers were required to keep track of and bring to the clinic for updating at the time of the visit. Family planning clients had their own cards that they, too, brought to the clinic. In this way clients, using multiple types of services, were tracked in an effort to coordinate care.

The reports do not mention a rich network of traditional healers in Cité Soleil. Among them were dozens of bonesetters and leaf doctors. Bernard et al. (1993) found in his ethnographic study of Cité Soleil ten different *hounfò-vodou* temples also used for healing purposes—where curative powers are derived principally from the *houngan* (priest) or *manbo* (priestess) who call on African ancestors for assistance. Haitian families rely heavily on medicinal herbal remedies for treating a variety of common illnesses (Rouzier 1998). These plants can be purchased relatively easily in the open markets. In my own sample of practitioner interviews, I spoke at length with two *doktè fèy* or leaf doctors and one houngan, all of whom shared with me their treatment style and the types of abortifacients, side-effect remedies, and family planning "methods" they prescribed. Many women (including clients from the family planning center) use the services of a doktè fèy with varying success. The utility of these practitioners is elaborated on in the final chapter of this book.

Given this relatively sophisticated health care system within this slum community, why are the poor so sick, and how is this linked to high fertility? Although health is considered a priority within individuals' urban survival strategy, accessing it and paying for it are nearly insurmountable obstacles. Because Haiti's health care system is generally based on fee for service (Auguste 1995), access to health services is directly related to economic power.

The Many Costs of Family Planning

In the Cité Soleil family planning center, birth control methods were supplied at what program planners call a "small" cost to the client. In 1993, birth control methods were priced as follows: condom (Hg 1), pills (Hg 1), IUD (Hg 15), injectables (Hg 5), and Norplant (Hg 15). Population planners in Haiti insist that when clients are asked to pay for a method, they consider it more valuable. Large-scale national survey results showed that indeed women and men report that they would be willing to pay for a method (CHI/CDC 1991), but in in-depth interviews all of the participants said that they wished they did not have to pay.[4] Looking at the implication of user fees for women's health care utilization in several African countries, Nanda (2002:127) notes that "lack of access to resources and inequitable decision-making power mean that when poor women face out-of-pocket costs such as user fees, the cost of health care may become out of reach." Nanda argues for "hard evidence" of the impact of user fees on women's health outcomes and reproductive health services, as well as a need to explain "how women cope with health care costs and what trade-offs they make in order to pay for health care" (2002:133). Studies in Zaire, Ghana, and Tanzania, all cited in Nanda's work, indicate that charging user fees does not always accompany improvements in the quality of care or availability of medications.

Haitian women were quick to provide more hard evidence regarding user fees. They explained that no cost was a "small" cost. Once the initial fee was charged, follow-up fees could be even more expensive, particularly when they entailed treating side effects related to method use, seeking other laboratory procedures requested by the physician, or purchasing antibiotics for STIs. The cost of these treatments, as detailed during clinical encounters, could easily wipe out an entire household.

But family planning care in the center also had hidden direct costs. The Hg 5 paid by injectable users, who are also asked to purchase their syringe, could pay for a small can of tomato paste, enough to use in two meals, or a small can of Carnation milk for a hungry baby. All of these costs required of women clients are relatively heavy financial burdens. Weighed against the urgent need to pay the rent or prepare a meal for a hungry family, the long-term "benefits" of family planning quickly lose their value. Poverty in Cité Soleil reduces choices to the short term. The costs and benefits of seeking treatment are weighed scrupulously against other immediate competing needs, including water and food.

Added to the direct costs of purchasing a contraceptive method and successfully staying on the method are the indirect costs of related reproductive health conditions.[5] Since the family planning center was the main place for women to address their reproductive concerns and the only center not run by the nuns, some women came to the clinic worried about method failure and possible pregnancy. In such cases, women were asked to purchase a pregnancy test first (an expensive request) and then return with the result. In the event of an unintended pregnancy, options for ending a pregnancy are rarely safe and certainly not cheap. In a recent study of abortion knowledge, attitudes, and practice in Haiti, Haitian researchers confirmed that abortions and attempted abortions are widespread. In a nationally representative sample, a significant number of women confirmed having had at least one abortion: 46 percent (of 1,563 women) responding to the individual interviews and 65 percent (of 64 women) who participated in in-depth discussion groups. A small minority indicated they had at least three abortions (TAG 2001).

If in need of an abortion, women from Cité Soleil would generally resort to traditional methods because they were cheaper and easier to access than medical alternatives. Abortions are illegal in Haiti except in the case of rape or incest. In such cases, legal permission is required of the client; however, accessing the "judicial system" in Haiti is impossible for poor women. Over half of the community sample said that once they knew they were pregnant, they tried all sorts of different combinations of abortifacients either prescribed by community leaf doctors or purchased in local markets. Some efforts included a cola douche immediately following intercourse or boiled parsley tea with salt, imbibed with large quantities of *grenn kamoken* (quinine pills, generally used as antimalarials)—three dozen pills, reported in one case. In many instances women were extremely sick following these regimes, some of which are known to be highly toxic. If these methods failed, then modern methods were used. One doctor who worked in the family planning center in the late 1980s performed abortions on the side as part of his own private practice. He charged approximately Hg 300 (about twenty days of factory labor), a cost that was out of reach for most poor women. Another woman interviewed indicated that she received *plizyè piki* (many shots) from a Port-au-Prince doctor who probably induced abortion with high doses of Depo-Provera.

In Cité Soleil, other hidden indirect costs of seeking birth control include the reallocation of time and resources within the household and the community. In Haiti, women have primary responsibility for the health of the household. This requires cash for health maintenance—and children's needs usually come first. Additionally, similar to what Nanda (2002) found in a study in Uganda, when a household member is sick, the burden of care falls on women, and this in turn chisels away at their potential earning time, thus making the purchase of health care or a family planning method an even more remote possibility.

Babette, a family planning promoter in Cité Soleil, provides an example of how deleterious sickness in a household can be. Babette had worked at the family-planning center for five years. She was scrupulous about not missing work, until her husband fell ill with HIV. In order to continue her work, she had to have a child at home to care for her ailing husband. Rather than pull her son from school, she asked Katusky, her eldest daughter, to stay home. This seemed like a relatively easy solution, but in order to fulfill her duties at home, Katusky had to stop selling in the market. Bereft of Katusky's marketing income, Babette needed to invest in a home-based business—one that Katusky could tend to while taking care of her father. When her husband died, she sold an old suitcase, radio, and a dresser to help pay for his funeral. To this day she claims that she has not been able to reestablish the precarious economic balance that she had lost while caring for her ill partner and family.

Whether due to direct or indirect costs, paying for health care services is deeply challenging in the Haitian context. The cost of paying for family planning, although seemingly scant, proved to be a deterrent to some users and insurmountable to most. "Costs" are regularly debated at the level of the experts—cost containment, cost recovery, cost efficiency, cost effectiveness. Tellingly, an author of an interim family planning evaluation from USAID argued, "There is very little common understanding of [these] relevant terms" and "There is near universal misunderstanding of concepts associated with 'sustainability'" (USAID 1993:51). In the same document, USAID consultants evaluating the private-sector family planning project noted that fee-for-service initiatives and "other revenue generating measures" should be investigated as a potential way to support the high costs of providing family planning services in Haiti. Not once in the entire report was the cost borne by clients considered or mentioned. On the contrary, the report suggested finding ways to have the poor shoulder even more costs.

Why is it that the provision of basic contraceptive supplies, pregnancy tests, and antibiotics to treat widespread STIs are not covered as part of family-planning services? Whenever I posed this question to the personnel at USAID, the issue of "excessive costs" always surfaced. Readers will recall that per capita expenditure for family planning in Haiti is twice that of any other country in the hemisphere. Sustainability of public health projects in the Haitian context, Farmer (2002:2) argues, is indeed gravely misunderstood—and misappropriated. Addressing the general lack of commitment to pay for HIV retroviral treatment for the world's poor, Farmer's arguments could just as pointedly address the provision of contraceptive methods.

> What's our excuse, after almost a decade of experience with antiretrovirals? We can blame the high cost of pharmaceuticals or shrug and point to the manifestly weak health infrastructures in such settings. But if we are honest, we will conclude that our own ambivalence regarding HIV therapy for the poorest has hamstrung comprehensive efforts as much as anything else. It may be assumed that naturally conservative funders, looking for consensus and "safe bets," would be unlikely to pay for such projects if they are so contested within the very community charged with promoting the health of the globe's poor.

Indeed, passing the burden of paying more for family planning services to clientele seemed like an immoral suggestion in the context of the poverty that gripped the community. And yet USAID stated that the policy "in Haiti is that all products [contraceptives] should become self-financing after 5 years" (USAID 1993).

Because they kalkile, almost every day and all the time, Haitians are well aware of what is required to access health care or avoid an unintended pregnancy. A group of women activists reflecting on these "costs" addressed this very same issue, but cast it in more political terms: "The State must revoke the tax on medicine, and it must place controls on the price of medicines. In a little country which is so poor and where there are so many health problems, the state should not allow pharmacies to make a 33 percent profit on medicines. Illness is not a business" (Caritas of Haiti 1986:4).

This desire for affordable and accessible health care was even more sharply articulated through the community's political activism.

The Politics of Health Care: 1986–1996

Although the majority of the poor in Cité Soleil were excluded from economic power, this rarely stopped their determination to organize for political power. Prior to the collapse of the Duvalier dictatorship, most organizing was underground. With the ousting of Baby Doc in 1986, the political landscape transformed radically. Popular organizations took to the streets of Cité Soleil. Their demands, reflected in popular organizing activities, were premised on access to basic human rights: fair access to food and water, education, work, and health care. Since CDS had such a prominent role in the community, demands for improving life often centered on the community's health care system. The impact of popular organizations' challenging "development" efforts in Cité Soleil was substantial. Like the activities described in Paley's (2001) work in Chile during the Pinochet regime, Haitian popular organizations increasingly engaged in critical analyses of the way the country's political economy affected people's health.

During 1986 and 1987, the populace of Cité Soleil had little tolerance for any remnant of the injustice that they had suffered under the Duvaliers. There was a feeling that, at last, they might matter. Gunshots filled the air night and day, and curfews were imposed. Tonton makout-s (armed militias) who previously lived in Cité Soleil went into hiding in the countryside. One day in July 1987, a makout attempted to return, but he was spotted within minutes. Viewing the scene from a two-story building on rue du Soleil, I saw huge swarms of people seemingly consume him. The CDS general director rushed to quell the scene. He was, in fact, spending an increasing amount of time suppressing political battles in the community. When he was unable to control the situation, the military was called in; they beat and arrested several Cité Soleil residents and rescued the makout. Everything was tenuous in Haiti. There was still little justice, but what was different was that the poor felt they could finally make demands.

In the midst of this popular demand for greater political participation, CDS became the center of controversy. CDS managed the family planning center, among other health services, and was perceived as having total control of community activities and services. CDS's well-known links to international aid and a long line of visiting foreign researchers, seen as part of the international economy of Haiti, added to the controversy. It is public information that CDS was said to have received upwards of $14 million U.S. dollars, a large part of this from USAID, for health and development projects in major urban areas throughout the country since the mid-1980s—a figure far higher than payments to any single ministry in the government (Marquez 1995). That the organization built its political clout on the battles fought in the name of public health did not sit well with the populace, since they were no healthier for it.

In an effort to control the increasingly discontented and vocal citizenry, the CDS began "buying up" residents and groups, promising them money and jobs if they would cooperate with CDS efforts in the community. CDS paid selected health-care workers and promoters "bonuses," with the understanding that they should report to him about disturbances within the neighborhoods. One family planning promoter who acted as an informant to the director suddenly appeared at work in beautiful clothes, with painted fingernails and adorned in gold jewelry. That this "promotion" did not need to be hidden speaks to the power that CDS had over this community and the residents. She was also seen reporting to the CDS on a regular basis. Her work as a family planning promoter continued, even though she was observing and reporting information far beyond the normal reproductive health data that she was trained to gather. A poor woman herself, she embodied the way in which international agencies and their local representatives exploit the poor to serve their own ends. Her behavior did not go unnoticed in the community.

Apart from singling out specific health care workers, CDS also supported selected local organizations as a means of maintaining political leverage. One such organization was KPDSS (Komite pou devlopman Site Solèy), the Committee for the Development of Cité Soleil. Although a deplorable community by most standards, Cité Soleil was almost always among the sites visited by foreign diplomats, high-level officials, and major international assistance donors, whose itineraries often included a staged tour of the local medical programs and clinics.[6] These visitors often met with several grassroots groups, who performed skits and songs about their liberty and health. These encounters with selected community groups were part of an effort to show visiting diplomats why USAID was so pleased with CDS, its local nonprofit organization. KPDSS allegedly received funds directly from Marilyn Quayle during her brief diplomatic visit in July 1991 (GRAIP 1994). Thus, allegiances to CDS usually paid off in one way or another.

Contesting Health Care and Quenching the "Thirst"

But the majority of groups and their members, especially the most vocal ones, could not be bought. What Marilyn Quayle did not see or hear were the other political activists in Cité Soleil: those raising questions about how health care was delivered to the poor. One such organization was OLS (Operasyon Leve Solèy), Operation Uplift [Cité] Soleil. In the mid to late 1980s, OLS members met regularly in one of the Cité's oldest neighborhoods and were closely aligned with other politically progressive poor people. When OLS was founded, one of its primary goals was to raise questions about the function and existence of CDS. Many OLS members were actually former CDS health-care workers who had protested working conditions and low pay and were subsequently told to leave. After being fired, they turned to political organizing.

Robert, twenty-one years old and an OLS organizer, described the organization's history.

When OLS was founded, there were about 500 members, which was in March 1989. Before 1986, when Duvalier was still in power, there was a similar movement, but we centered our work on cleaning our neighborhood, improving our living conditions, but our work was underground.

When Duvalier left, in 1986, we were joyful. It was only after he left that we began to really understand the degree to which we suffered. Everybody, even the children, got involved in what we called "neighborhood politics," in our neighborhoods, in the tight little corridors where we live all cramped up.

OLS organizing during the post-Duvalier period was impressive. Among their goals was to teach the poor, young and old, to read.[7] Literacy schools flourished in Cité Soleil with the help of the progressive wing of the Catholic Church and the political motivation provided by popular organizations. Another popular organizer said this: "The work of literacy was important. The people learned to speak about not only what was good in our society but also what needed to change, and that's when our problems began. Father Volel, well, he used to encourage us, but when it was clear that the popular will was surfacing, he came and threw us out of the school where we were learning. *Baow!* Like that!"

This did not stop OLS or other organizations from their work; now firmly entrenched, they educated and informed the masses through community meetings and home visits. Their organization served as an institutional base, albeit informal, for the poor. Learning to read bolstered organizers and helped them place their own experiences of the unjust economic structure in Haiti within a more regional and global context. As they read about Nicaragua and Brazil, where literacy campaigns had transformed the political landscape, new things seemed possible. *Pèp la te swaf pou sa* (the people were thirsty for that), reflected an OLS leader.

Janine, a woman who was actively involved with OLS, put the issue of this thirst for literacy into a historical framework: "Under France we were diminished while they filled their coffers. Today the upper classes still speak French and act superior. They don't want us to read, because they know if we learn to read, we won't be their slaves, we won't be their maids and servants any more, and we won't work in their factories for just a few cents. When you can read, you know your rights. This is why the mass of people can't read."

Since many of the leaders of this movement had once worked with CDS as community health workers, their experience with community-based delivery of health care services was intimate. OLS members utilized their knowledge to address what they perceived as injustice by educating people about their rights in the health care system, particularly with regard to family planning. When clinical trials were performed without explanation or when clients were asked to pay for medical supplies in the midst of large-scale starvation, they questioned how international public health funds were being spent. Another young leader said,

> We took our experiences as community health workers and applied them. We helped the people see why they were still unhealthy, even though Cité Soleil had so many health care facilities. We explained the process: how CDS had many organizations supporting it, including USAID, and how thoroughly it was funded, and how we—the population of Cité Soleil—had no voice in this process. It is on the backs of the poor that they receive this money and yet we are silenced. We revolted [and] we mobilized in fourteen different neighborhoods in Cité Soleil. Our job was to motivate people, to teach them about what was happening. The people began to see clearly and our organization grew.

Within less than two years of the Duvalier ouster, political organizing around health care became a potent force within this community. OLS questioned—in no small way—the workings of international aid. In spite of a series of dictators and regimes that moved in and out of power from 1986 to 1990, the poor in Cité Soleil stayed focused on their demands. Health, they argued, is a human right. At one point I explained to a high official in the Health, Population, and Nutrition division of USAID that there was considerable and growing dissent among the poor in Cité Soleil regarding USAID-funded health services. The official was quick to snap, "There is no possible way that those people in Cité Soleil understand that we [USAID] give CDS money. Come on! They don't know how international aid works!"

Second-Hand Family Planning: 1987–1989

The CDS family planning center was part of the controversy over health care in this community for several reasons. First, residents long understood that thousands of U.S. dollars were being spent on a clinic, and yet the services inevitably made the users sick with side effects. Second, men, who already felt threatened because their partners might be using contraceptives in secret, were vehemently opposed to longer-lasting methods, such as injectable contraceptives. Women, on the other hand, liked this method for the very reason that they could use it without their partners' knowing. Injectable contraceptives (Depo Provera) rank among the most popular methods, along with oral contraceptives. Third, the care provided to clients was deficient. Little emotional support or privacy, differences in language and culture between health professionals and their clients, and a disrespectful medical staff were among the concerns cited by the community (Maternowska 1986; Maynard-Tucker 1991).

In 1987, CDS initiated its family-planning promoter program in an effort to boost the poor clinic statistics. In conjunction with women from the community, I designed and implemented this program, using CDS as the institutional base for funding purposes. Through a grant from a Washington, D.C.–based nonprofit organization—separate from CDS or USAID—the program was initiated with six women promoters. Prior to this, community health workers were responsible for primary health care tasks, including family planning, though family planning was the lowest priority among their tasks and so received little, if any, attention during home visits.

The program, which sought to empower health care workers, namely, poor and illiterate women from the community, was not without problems. There was enormous controversy around the educational materials produced for this program. Although they were targeted to an audience with low literacy rates, designed in collaboration with the community and a Haitian artist, and were qualitatively tested and assessed, the materials were never fully utilized. USAID population division officials attempted to ban the materials, in spite of the fact that they were popular in poor communities around the country. The health officer stated that they were "obscene and bordering on pornography" and that "they did not appeal to the white collar in Haiti." During an initial training session in 1987, while I was teaching promoters how to use health literacy booklets, the military raided the classroom, confiscated my notes and cassettes, and disbanded the meeting.

The next week, at the request of the undaunted promoters-in-training, the work was resumed. The family planning promoters were trained and prepared to educate women and men, encouraging community members to visit the CDS family planning center. The promoters became so skilled that they were asked to train other promoters around the country. Although the promoters were never given the respect they deserved—and were often not paid during times of serious economic scarcity—they continued to work with the family planning center. Family planning statistics improved minimally during this period (Despagne 1988). The promoter program brought family planning activities into the heart of the community.

Later that year, an acceptability study for Norplant began (Kane et al. 1990). Norplant is made of plastic capsules or silicone rods implanted under the skin that release hormones slowly over five years. Cité Soleil was named as one of three research sites in Haiti. These trials were observed closely, since there was much hope among the staff, as well as the population experts in Haiti and the United States, that this method might provide a boost to the community's poor family planning record. Clients were somewhat hesitant about any new methods. Women who eventually entered the study told me they did so because they wanted a method that would not "cause so many problems." Posters about Norplant adorned the clinic walls and women began to ask for information. The potential for a method that, once inserted, would protect a woman against pregnancy for five years seemed like a feasible solution to high dropout rates at the clinic. Additionally, for women who traveled to the countryside, Norplant seemed like a sensible solution, since follow-up was supposed to be minimal. The only caveat was that a woman needed to return to her original provider to have the device removed.

As a regular in the clinic, I was able to observe all stages of the research. The first step, consent, proved disconcerting. The consent form was prepared in French and was exceedingly long. After being given only a brief and partial verbal translation into Creole, clients who agreed to what they were told were physically guided to sign the form (partly because they could neither read nor write). Throughout the trials, standards of care were low, certainly in comparison to research I have participated in at my own university. In addition to minimizing clients' complaints, the clinic physicians were generally intolerant when side effects were mentioned. Side effects from Norplant typically mentioned by clients included nausea, dizziness, headaches, and irregular bleeding. Because of these side effects and often infections at the site of the implant, some women returned to the clinic and insisted on having the implants removed. The right to request removal, buried within the consent form, was met with considerable scorn.

One hot afternoon a woman arrived with an infection in her arm where the Norplant had been inserted. She claimed she could no longer lift heavy loads onto her head, an economic liability for a Haitian market woman. After several attempts by the doctor and nurse to dissuade her from removing the device, the doctor bellowed out to me, "She's so stupid—look at her, she asked to have this put in and now what—take it out?" He proceeded to remove the implant, buried deep inside an infected area in her upper arm, despite pained responses from the woman indicating that the local anesthetic had not yet taken effect. It was later recognized by experts that indeed the capsules tend to migrate in the arm, and finding them can be very difficult, making clients prone to scarring and sometimes nerve damage.

Above all, the family planning service infrastructure was below standard for carrying out the Norplant research. When services do not meet basic standards, clients suffer. Conditions in other areas in Haiti where Norplant trials were also carried out made what happened in Cité Soleil seem benign. At a hospital in Léogane, Haiti, the American clinic director there told Canham-Clyne and Cooley-Prost (1996:4) that women requesting implant removals had to go through a series of "education" sessions.[8] "If, on a second or third visit, a woman insists, the implant will be removed. However, unless the clinic staff determines that she "has a serious medical problem" she is charged a fee of Hg 80 [US$30] for removal within the first two years—even though AID provides it free and the fee constitutes some 20 percent of the average Haitian annual income."

According to the investigators, the American clinic director later defended this practice saying, "Norplant is expensive. USAID and the program have made a significant investment in these women" (Canham-Clyne and Cooley-Prost 1996:4). To its credit, CDS did not institute the practice of charging women for removal of the method. The general director of the CDS firmly denounced the use of such fees. However, CDS hired special Norplant recruiters during the study. As such, study recruits may have been heavily persuaded to use Norplant over other methods, diminishing a woman's right to choose from several methods in an unbiased way.

Women in the community challenged the terms of this research. Activists in the community brought several popular organizations together and challenged the medical system head-on. Members of a Haitian women's advocacy group from New York interviewed women and health-care workers in Haiti (Canham-Clyne and Cooley-Prost 1996). Soon after, a published booklet surfaced: *Norplant (R): "Piki 5 an Planing Familyal Pèpè Nan Peyi Dayiti"* (NORPLANT: The Five Year Method—Cast-off Family Planning in the Country of Haiti).[9] It detailed alarming ethical and research concerns. Consent, follow-up treatment for side effects, and problems with removal were among the issues noted (Koalisyon 28 Jiye Chalmay Peral 1991). Community organizers used the book to educate.

In spite of this evidence, neither the clinic nor the donor community paid heed to what Norplant clients were saying. An entirely different interpretation was coming from USAID, where program evaluators said, "The method is well-suited to the Haitian environment and is in high demand in spite of virtually no marketing" (USAID 1993:ii). Not long after the booklet's publication, USAID "successfully negotiated" with AID/Washington to make Haiti the largest USAID-funded Norplant program worldwide. Not surprisingly, increasingly negative opinions began to surface where family planning activities were promoted.

Numerous legal issues around the use of Norplant surfaced during the decade that followed FDA approval in 1990, and shipments to clinics in the United States were suspended by the year 2000. On September 13, 2000, the FDA issued a statement advising patients who had implants inserted after October 20, 1999 to contact their doctors about using a nonhormonal backup method. On July 26, 2002, Wyeth Pharmaceuticals, in conjunction with the FDA, released a statement that it will no longer produce Norplant due to "limitations in product component supplies" (UCSF 2003). Norplant is still used in many, though not all, clinics throughout Haiti.

Giving Voice to the Victory: 1990–1991

In 1990, Haiti's political landscape was again transformed when the then liberation theology priest, Jean-Bertrand Aristide, who had actively worked with the poor in Cité Soleil, became the popular candidate in the country's first democratic election. It was rumored and later substantiated (in a BBC documentary) that CDS had paid "volunteers"—the special family planning promoters among them—to campaign in the same elections for the favored U.S.-backed candidate Marc Bazin, a former World Bank economist, although to little avail. Kim Ives (1995:45), a longtime reporter of Haitian events, captured it well: "Despite the money Bazin distributed throughout the country in an attempt to buy votes and the $36 million spent on his campaign, thousands of Haitians poured into the streets during Aristide's gigantic campaign rallies shouting *Li pa lajan, non se volontè, wi* (I'm not here for money, it's my free will).

At least 95 percent of Cité Soleil residents voted for the priest, endearingly called Titid. Residents lined up at daybreak, well before the polls opened. His victory was a landslide around the country, garnering 67 percent of the national vote. With the election of President Aristide, the nation watched a slow shift in government priorities from the elite to the masses and from nonparticipatory to participatory. Even if symbolic, this gave a needed boost to the many social movements in Cité Soleil. The transformation of political power from above shifted the strategies of the community's social movements to focus on increasingly political demands. Similar in nearly identical ways to Paley's (2001) account of a grassroots health care movement in post-dictatorship Chile, OLS members began to examine the *konjonkti politik* (the political circumstances) critically and the effects and forms of power operating in their lives.

Almost immediately after the election, on December 16, 1990, health organizers felt free to voice their concerns. Graffiti began appearing all over the walls of the community and even on the barrier walls of the USAID complex down the road (though it was quickly covered with fresh paint), *Aba USAID! Pa fè kòb sou tet pòv!* (Down with USAID! Stop making money on the heads of the poor!). OLS focused much of their critique on the president of CDS and the organization's ability to garner public health contracts through USAID. CDS's work with several U.S. universities was not widely accepted by residents. This discontent was fueled by the fact that there were multiple clinical trials and investigative research projects ongoing at the center. Residents maintained that they were not fully informed about these studies or their own health status once enrolled in the studies. The phrase *nou se kobay* (we are guinea pigs) was often repeated to me.

The majority of studies were conducted on pregnant women or women in their reproductive years. A sample of research topics includes: HIV and women of reproductive years (Boulos et al. 1990; Boulos et al. 1991; Halsey et al. 1990; Halsey et al. 1992; Markham et al. 1994), sexually transmitted diseases (Boulos et al. 1992), sexual behavior (Halsey et al. 1992), general family planning (Boulos, Pierre-Louis, and Tafforeau 1986), Norplant (Kane et al. 1990), IUD use (Jacob 1987), condoms (Boulos et al. 1991), Depo-Provera (Tafforeau, Allman, and Allman 1985; Tafforeau and Boulos 1986), breast milk (Dowell et al. 1993), and measles (Halsey 1993; Holt et al. 1993).

The Norplant study, coupled with the series of clinical studies using pregnant women or their children as "participants," was deeply problematic for the poor. Clinical and acceptability trials came to symbolize the organizational control over basic human services and rights that OLS and other groups were fighting to reverse. Although popular organizations consistently questioned CDS activities, it was not until 1991 that they began to contest in large public demonstrations what CDS did, and failed to do, for the overall health of the community. One organizer of OLS offered stated, "We all felt that they [CDS] were not really working with the community the way they should have been. Everything they did, even food aid, became a political tool. CDS kept getting more and more power and more and more financing. We were tired of it. At one point we closed [the president of CDS] out of Cité Soleil because we weren't getting the health services that were mandated."

The most hostile act against the CDS health services and family planning activities occurred in January 1991, during an attempted coup against Aristide, led by a former tonton makout seeking to reverse the people's democratic choice. In an act of protest against the coup, a countrywide *dechoukaj* (uprooting) of elitist symbols of wealth occurred. Crowds attacked rich storeowners in downtown Port-au-Prince and burned and gutted their boutiques. The Catholic cathedral was also vandalized, in symbolic protest against the Catholic Church hierarchy's public denouncements of President Aristide.[10] CDS offices were not spared in the pillaging. Groups of residents ransacked the headquarters, destroying computers, shredding files, and breaking into supplies.

Later, in August 1991, a concert was organized in Cité Soleil where the country's most outspoken political singer and later mayor of Port-au-Prince, Manno Charlemagne, performed a politically satirical performance. The poor in Cité Soleil adored Manno for his songs about injustice. One of these, an apparently impromptu tune, concerned the family planning center as just another "tool" for the CDS complex, with particular reference to injectables: "and what they use on dogs in the United States and give to our women here," and later how women in Haiti were "guinea pigs for the five year method [Norplant]."[11]

Silence through Violence: September 30, 1991

During the Aristide government's brief first period in power, land reform commenced, literacy campaigns took hold again, and a judicial system was initiated.[12] From the perspective of OLS and other agents of change at the community level, these were the political and social measures required to address poverty *and* its associated high fertility. OLS continued to question how CDS operated. Elsewhere in Haitian society, notably among the elite, such massive structural reforms were not well accepted. Aristide's government was overthrown on September 30, 1991, when seven months into his term a violent coup erupted. Aristide himself survived after being held hostage for some time, and was later whisked out of the country to Venezuela and then the United States. A de facto military government, headed by General Raoul Cédras, took over (Goff 2000).

As the political and economic situation worsened, following the post–coup d'état era in 1992, so, too, did the changing mechanisms of power and resistance both in the clinic and the community. The more residents contested their dwindling health care options, the more they were repressed. The price of such overt political organizing throughout Cité Soleil would now be paid. The military's main goal was to keep the people, especially those who believed in democracy, in fear. Members of the Revolutionary Front for the Advancement and Progress of Haiti (FRAPH)—also called *attaché-s*—the savage paramilitary group that was responsible for a prolonged wave of killings, rapes, and other atrocities—was the central source of violence in Cité Soleil. FRAPH was said to work in close cooperation with the Haitian army and often served as a front for the army (Nairn 1994, Grann 2001). The terror FRAPH inflicted was widespread. Thousands of Cité Soleil residents were displaced—seeking shelter from arrests, torture, and beating—and hundreds more were assassinated in raids on the community. Prominent leaders, some of them from OLS and associated movements, were killed in broad daylight, their faces completely cut out by machetes to impede identification. Everyone was silenced, but only temporarily. To survive, organizers moved *anba fey*—"underneath the leaves" (underground)—again.

The work of the family planning promoters, the few from CDS who actually remained employed during these hard times, was exceedingly risky. Solange, a patient and kind family planning promoter who had worked at the center since 1987, was visibly shaken one day after work: "Our work is much more difficult now. You go into a house and you don't know what you can say, you don't know who's listening. I've been asked to leave by men who I know were members of FRAPH—and I had to leave, because they could easily hit me or beat me. There was a time when almost all of the men were FRAPH. We were frightened; they didn't want anyone coming into the house, especially to talk about family planning, because it concerned women."

Association with CDS was an equally threatening prospect. Solange stated, "We would enter the house and we would say, 'Hello, we are the promoters for family planning from CDS,' and they would say 'Oh! We don't need family planning. Where's our food from CDS?' It scared us because we knew they were confusing us for the spies who were working all over the Cité as FRAPH. Of course it was dangerous."

At the end of our conversation Solange summed up sickness and politics in the same way that several of the community's residents did when I asked them about prioritizing sickness: *N ap mouri nan maladi prezidan* (We're dying from the president's sickness), which in the context of their suffering meant simply a slow and painful death from the lack of democracy.

By early 1993, in the midst of the three-year coup d'état carnage, undaunted political organizers came forth and noted that several of the community's more famous tonton makout-s, now members of FRAPH, began working in the CDS medical complex. Residents in interviews offered more evidence to back what political activists were reporting: that in addition to noting fertility and immunization status, these selected health agents were also keeping tabs on political affiliations and activities. It is said that information leading to attacks on pro-Aristide neighborhoods, and on specific individuals, was garnered during these "public health" surveys. Certain neighborhoods were demarcated as *Titid rèd* (thick with Aristide supporters). Many OLS organizers and members were among the targeted victims of violence. Dozens, if not hundreds, of residents claimed that they were denied primary health care services if it was clear that they were Aristide supporters.

One woman, ill with tuberculosis, recounted a visit to St. Catherine's, the CDS hospital. "They looked at me, asked me what neighborhood I lived in and told me to go home. We are suffering." While some received care, many did not. Water and food handouts from the nuns were also selective. McFadyen (1995:155–156) from the North American Congress on Latin America offered evidence of how poor infrastructure, compounded by political interests, served to punish the poor.

> No one disputes the fact that CDS was providing a useful service. It's only in the broader context that its potentially pernicious effects became apparent. Because the clinics could not possibly provide full health services for everyone, a selection process was inevitable. "The poor who are compliant and docile get health services," explained Gerard Blot, a progressive doctor who is familiar with CDS. "Those who are militant have trouble getting services." A select hundred malnourished babies were showered with attention and care, but what about the thousands of other impoverished children in the slum?

At the time, all of these allegations against CDS were dismissed—by almost everyone—as conspiracy theory. Later, in 1994, a string of journalists began to take the allegations seriously (LaRamée 1994; McFadyen 1995; NACLA 1994; Ridgeway 1994). Allan Nairn (1994), a seasoned reporter from *The Nation*, reported incriminating evidence that indeed CDS was using FRAPH members to perform so-called public health work with insidious and sometimes deadly results. The local warlord, who was the declared leader of FRAPH, Emmanuel "Toto" Constant, was later identified as a paid informant of the United States Central Intelligence Agency (CIA) (Grann 2001; Human Rights Watch 2002). Government sources later confirmed the claim that the CIA provided Constant with financial and strategic assistance (Concannon 2002; Grann 2001). In 2001, Toto Constant was convicted in absentia of murder for his involvement in a massacre in Haiti in 1994. Today he lives and works in Queens. Grann (2001) concludes that Constant's ties with U.S. intelligence may help to explain why Constant has not been returned to Haiti to face justice.

Fire, Politics, and Health Care Revisited: 1993–1996

Political repression was thick in the community and took on many guises in this period. In a symbolic move, to associate FRAPH with the former Duvalier

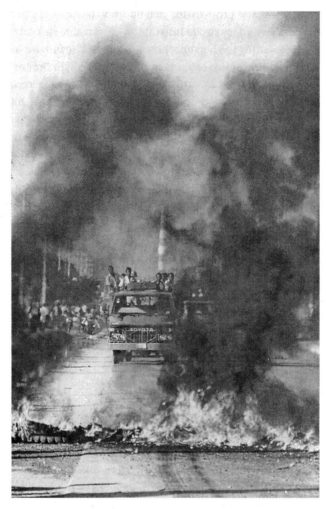

Route Nationale #1, 1994

dictatorship, the attachés in December of 1993 incited a campaign to reverse the name of the community from Cité Soleil back to Cité Simone, after François Duvalier's wife. To enforce this, attachés shot the tires of tap tap-s that had not replaced their "Cité Soleil" placards (identifying the terminus) with "Cité Simone." Evenings were just as hazardous as days. Even in sleep, the poor were vulnerable to attack. It was a time when the common inquiry of asking a person if they slept well was responded to like this: "Thanks to God, I got up. I'm here."

This once desperately avoided and rarely mentioned slum hit its peak of notoriety in December 1993, when a fire broke out in Soley 17, in an act reminiscent of the community's first urban planning exercise when houses were cleared (Associated Press 1993a; *Time* 1994). Soley 17 was one of the community's most politically active and pro-Aristide neighborhoods. Accounts of this disaster indicated that the military strode into Cité Soleil at II a.m. carrying grenades, guns, and gasoline, setting the neighborhood in flames. The fire was in apparent retaliation for the killing of two soldiers by a Cité Soleil mob. Dozens of people died or "disappeared" during the attack—and many of these were small children. Estimates of how many people lost their homes were as high as ten thousand (McFadyen 1995). Few know for sure what really happened, though residents claim that stories of "attacks against the military" are commonly used as excuses to blame, punish, and silence the politically active poor. Representatives from CDS were there to witness the fire shortly after flames broke out. State functionaries later noted that 1,053 families lost their homes in the flames, and up to fifty people died. Angry residents claim that the people who started the fire—FRAPH—were the same people who worked inside CDS and were handing out aid after the fire (Marquez 1995). The fire served its purpose and sent a warning, reminding the poor of who remained in control.

When Angélique Kidjo's jazzy African voice crooned over the radio, the residents of Cité Soleil were reminded of the many fires they had endured, which explained that wry smile on their faces. The lyrics, in this setting, made great sense.

> Fire burns in our hearts, fire burns in our houses.
> They say it's for reasons of the state.
> They say it's in the name of justice.
> Today torturers are everywhere: Tomorrow who will judge them?
> Fire burns in our hearts, fire burns in our houses.

Reconstruction on the site did not begin until two years later, in 1995, even though the U.S. Embassy gave $100,000 to CDS as aid for the homeless in 1993 (Associated Press 1993b). The construction of 162 houses was finally completed, but not until 1999. The Government of Haiti claimed it would distribute cash (Hg 2700 or US$180) to approximately thousand families who were identified as victims (Haiti Info 1999).

In October 1994, President Aristide, ousted for three years, returned to Haiti. With considerable fanfare, he was escorted by the U.S. military, which led to a prolonged five-year occupation. U.S. soldiers arriving in Haiti to oust the de facto dictatorship were told that FRAPH was a legitimate political party that needed to be respected and protected. In the intervention's first days, the U.S. Embassy arranged a press conference outside the presidential palace for Constant to announce his transition to politics. The conference was cut short because even a cordon of U.S. soldiers could not protect Constant from the enraged crowd. The last U.S. troops pulled out of Haiti in January 2000, marking the end of a five-year presence. When multinational forces first arrived in Haiti, it was rare to find their vehicles inside Cité Soleil, which left residents vulnerable, since many of the paramilitary thugs were at large and still armed. Later, military vehicles began entering the community. Popular will surfaced soon after, and U.S. military intervention and later the United Nations multinational forces provided considerably more security than had been provided in the previous three years.

The return of President Aristide, though more significantly the return of "democracy," gave way to massive rejuvenation of the popular movement and concomitantly the controversy surrounding health care. During an interview an organizer summed up the community's determination: *Nou p ap fè bak* (we're not going backward). Graffiti again exploded on the walls of Cité Soleil. "Down with [the CDS President]/[and] the families of the 30th September" (referring to the elite families who financed the coup d'état of 1991). Slogans supporting the popular organizations that had been terrorized during the three-year coup d'état regime also covered the walls. Demonstrations and speak-outs occurred, where hordes of local activists were anxious to tell international visitors and journalists about the terrorism in Cité Soleil, which they believed was controlled through the CDS medical complex.

CDS responded, on October 25, 1994, by temporarily shutting down all but one CDS clinic, including the family planning center. The closure of the CDS health network, contracted by USAID to provide services, lasted over a week. That same day a prominent popular organization, composed of a majority of OLS members, demanded to negotiate with the CDS president, who responded that he would not speak with *vakabon* (loosely translated as meaning, in this case, "totally reprehensible derelicts"). The divisions remained and the struggle continued.

Mintz (1974) once characterized the fundamental cleavage in Haitian society as one that had no unifying institutional forms capable of mediating or settling conflicts. He claimed at the time, and many other scholars of Haitian society have agreed, that "the will of the Haitian people is not heard by those who are content to rule." The returned President Aristide was no exception. In stunning contrast to the fiery antiestablishment rhetoric that characterized his speeches prior to the coup, he declared January 31, 1995, "Cité Soleil Day" and, on behalf of the government of Haiti, gave a $1.8 million check to CDS for rebuilding the area burned in December 1993 (Libète 1995a).

Residents skeptically denounced the pomp and circumstance surrounding the exchange of money. Women on the scene said that since their homes had been destroyed in the fire, they expected to be given new ones. However, the poor in Haiti rarely have legal title to land or property. Were they going to have to rent these houses? Were they going to have to purchase them? Were they guaranteed access to housing at all? As is usually the case in this community, no one told them anything.

Following this public event in Cité Soleil, the CDS president was physically attacked and his car windows smashed. The multinational force rescued him and arrested his attackers. That same day, in a familiar act of retaliation, all CDS health and nutrition centers were ordered shut down. They remained closed for a week. Popular organizers in Cité Soleil insisted that until they were actively involved in the design, implementation, maintenance, and evaluation of development projects in Cité Soleil, these projects would fail. Rebuilding houses without addressing issues of justice or legal rights neglected the pressing political demands of the poor. A community organizer, incensed by this, finished his interview with me rather eloquently by defining, from the residents' perspective, the concept of community participation: "CDS works in the community, not with the community. All we are asking is that they work with us, not against us. It's our right."

On October 15, 1995, during an official state visit to Haiti, Vice President Al Gore met with President Aristide in the palace. They discussed efforts to rebuild Haiti's democracy in an attempt to maintain stability. Meanwhile, Tipper Gore, the vice president's wife, was whisked off in an entourage of American Embassy officials, Haitian government representatives, and other VIPs to see the "sights" in Port-au-Prince.

As per protocol, prominent among these sights was CDS. The CDS officials were present to escort Mrs. Gore through the hospital, the malnutrition centers, the clinics, and the craft centers. She, like Marilyn Quayle, who received a similar tour in 1991, was undoubtedly impressed. After all, CDS was still USAID's favorite health project. The visit received considerable press, chiefly because at least one hundred protesters in Cité Soleil demonstrated against CDS by stoning the motorcade, shattering the windows of two cars and injuring a U.S. soldier. One of two vehicles stoned had as passengers Mrs. Gore's personal assistant, a White House photographer, and two doctors. Allegedly the CDS general director was among them. According to the *Washington Post*, "U.S. Officials said the protest appeared to be spontaneous, with Gore's motorcade getting caught in the middle of a local dispute between slum dwellers and the director of the U.S.-funded health center. Aid workers said residents of Cité Soleil believe that too little aid given to the center trickles down to the community and that money is siphoned off by administrators" (Marquez 1995:17).

Following the eruption, U.S. officials in Haiti said they were aware of the allegations against the CDS general director but had found no wrongdoing. Referring to these charges, a U.S. diplomat who spoke on condition of anonymity said, "The fact is we don't know. We are not an investigative agency. U.S. laws require that we give our grants on the basis of professional ability. People don't have to pass political correctness tests" (Marquez 1995:17).

In a press release, CDS noted that following the attack, residents in Cité Soleil burned vehicles and vandalized Cité Soleil buildings. Also noted were attacks on staff working in the CDS hospital and other aggressions by armed individuals from the community. Several organizers reminded me that the crowd did not have guns. Another organizer continued, "CDS does not want to respond to the real needs of the people. When they talk about the guns it is just so that USAID has reason to get out." The CDS general director asked the Haitian government for security support but to no avail (CDS 1996). On March 31, 1996, in what seemed to be the final form of retaliation, CDS permanently terminated its public health activities in the community (*Le Nouvelliste* 1996).

During the six-month period that followed, a series of troubled interactions between CDS, USAID, and the Ministry of Health ensued. When the CDS general director formally asked the Ministry of Health to take over its facilities and programs, the local dispute opened up a national and international debate about the ways that international aid agendas are determined, funded, and implemented. Arguments about Haiti's entire health care budget, including $27 million from the World Bank, were volleyed about at the same time. Although the ministry agreed it was their responsibility to "study" the problem and accommodate the new situation, the minister was clearly irritated. "We did not anticipate a budget for this center [CDS] because it did not belong to the ministry. One must understand the situation in which . . . [we] are placed . . . *and one should ask why*" (author's emphasis, Bohning 1996:21A).

Divisive arguments around who would fund and provide the community with health care soon surfaced: the ministry (with its strapped finances)? USAID? Or a new player, the World Bank? The ministry agreed to take over Cité Soleil *if* CDS finances were in order and problems with the local population were solved. But these stipulations were not well received by international donors, who were said "to be irritated with . . . the health ministry for what they saw as efforts to gain control over the . . . million[s]." According to Bohning (1996:21A), an investigative reporter for the *Miami Herald*, "So frustrated were donor agencies by the lack of cooperation from the health ministry that they drafted and delivered a joint 'informal note' to President Rene Préval in mid-March, warning that if they didn't get better cooperation, the money would be redirected to other countries."

The "warning" of losing funds altogether put the Haitian government in a decidedly weak position and unable to negotiate. In July 1996, the Ministry of Health, with USAID funding, resumed preventive and curative services for the residents of Cité Soleil, though on a greatly reduced scale. Family planning services, according to former clients, are *preske pa la* (almost nonexistent). Clearly unable to control the now internationally documented dissent and irreparably damaged relationship with the community, CDS and USAID had successfully passed the baton. USAID maintained full financial control of the health-care funds, ultimately ceding very little power to the Ministry of Health and, in the same act, absolved itself of direct care of this troubled community. The Haitian government, as is often the case, inherited a community health system they neither helped create nor participated in. In the end, they were left with a population of angry, violated, and ultimately sick people.

The Politicization of Health Care and the "Politics of Dependency"

This politicization of health care is now a common occurrence throughout the developing world. In Costa Rica, Morgan's (1993) work shows how bureaucrats implementing public health programs equated community participation with technological compliance. Yet Costa Ricans, like poor Haitians, associated the concept of community participation as a much broader activity, closely aligned with "democracy." As a community, Cité Soleil was caught in what Brodwin (1996:25) defines as "the current politics of dependency between Haitian institutions and international aid agencies," whereby the dominant class determines both the form of medicine and who has access to medical services. Added to this already complicated configuration of medicine and politics was the role of violence in Haiti. Exacerbated by aid institutions themselves, it pushed this conflict to an extreme. Mitchell (2002:153), writing about Egypt, notes that "Violence directed against people within a small community often relies on the power to impose silence. Victims disappear, survivors may fear to speak, investigations, if they occur, produce only accusations and hearsay, or are organized to serve larger political purposes. The original act of violence is therefore easily lost, and writing about it becomes an almost impossible effort to reconstruct events out of fragments and recover the voices of the missing."

In the case of Cité Soleil, accounts of violence focus on the violence of the poor and powerless, rather than violence used against them. In the process, scholarly accounts of political violence often end up being what Michael Taussig has called "the space of death"—an unaccounted-for void (quoted in Mitchell 2002). When people organize in Haiti, they often refer to needing *yon espas*, a space where organizing can happen. This space can be a physical space, a social space, or a broader political space. Although the "space of death" may loom large in Cité Soleil, it is unlikely ever to be fully silenced, but rather continually woven into a larger and more pressing struggle for basic human rights.

Health care in Cité Soleil became one of many repressive forces imposed on people's lives. In many ways the CDS public health strategy in this community mirrored local power structures that *chèf sèksyon* (rural sheriffs, vanguards of the tonton makout-s) once carried out in the countryside—small fiefdoms with little or no accountability and with complete control over community resources and entitlements. Attachés were agents reincarnating similar forms of power and terror. CDS claimed that its health services were based on community participation, but residents noted that this was not so. Residents' courage to challenge these so-called development interventions was a powerful and deeply menacing counterpoint to the fear and intimidation brought on by this "politic of dependency." When democracy flourished in Haiti, ever so briefly, participation became redefined as a threat to the power structures then in place. In Cité Soleil there remain several pervasive layers of political and economic control that permeate everyday existence in this community. Health rights are neither excluded nor immune from political manipulations.

Poor women and men indicate that reproduction is also deeply intertwined with their lack of rights and political will. Providing pills, injectable contraceptives, and condoms without addressing the structural causes of poverty and associated high fertility only deflects attention away from the real needs of the poor. A nurse who works closely with the poor puts the "problem of Haiti" and "problem of population control" in such a framework.

> It's not a problem of Haiti or of population control; it's a problem of social justice. It's a problem of social distribution, where the distribution of our country's resources is unequal. There is a tiny group who has every possibility to access their rights—by rights I mean the right to eat, the right to health care, the right to education, the right to live under a roof. Only a small number of people have these rights, because they have all the riches of the country in their hands and the majority, well, they live in what you see and smell here. So those people who are all concerned about family planning and how it will stop people from having children . . . in reality that's not what will resolve our problem.

Health care, as it was mandated by CDS, was not as benign as it purported to be. At best, the CDS program provided stopgap measures to very few health care problems while the social, economic, cultural, and political issues tied to residents' lives were never addressed. At worst, health care became a repressive apparatus used to control and silence—even physically repress—the political and health demands of the poor. The family-planning program that addressed "reproductive control" while ignoring the underlying causes of high fertility and poverty played a detrimental part in this process.

At the community level there were, and continue to be, far too many powerful forces working against potential contraceptive users. On one level, problems with side effects or method use were not just annoyances but potentially costly liabilities for poor women who could not afford or access the appropriate treatment they needed. On another level, community resistance, buried deep in political controversy and corruption, failed to reinforce women's decisions to use contraceptives. On the contrary, residents were discouraged from succumbing to a health system that denied people their health and human rights.

Rather than empowering clients through control of their reproduction, as family planning is so often touted as doing by development practitioners, the Cité Soleil family planning center actually prohibited the poor from broadening their base of power or gaining social support for their decision to use contraceptives. Taken one step further, the failure of family planning in this community is tantamount to collective resistance against an intervention that dominates the lives of the poor. Within this framework, rapid population growth results largely from efforts by the Haitian poor to cope and even revolt against their powerlessness in the face of the concentrated economic and political strength of the elite (Lappe and Schurman 1990). Resistance to using family planning reflects Haitians' lack of control and power experienced in the household, in the clinic, in the community and finally, as the next chapter shows, on the national and international scale.

6

The Political Economy of International Aid

Grounding Ethnography, Engaging History

Two kinds of rationality thus oppose each other: a substantive rationality which aims at a critical understanding of the world, and perhaps even critical action; and a formal or technical rationality, which understands the world in terms of technical solutions.

–Eric Wolf, *Reinventing Anthropology*

These days, a dusty sign swings in the hot sun outside the former CDS family planning clinic, it reads: Tribunal de Paix et Etat Civil de Cité Soleil (Peace and Marital Status Court). Still demographically relevant, though ironically so, this is now where local residents obtain birth, death, and marriage certificates. For a short period, family planning was available in a different place through the Ministry of Health's clinic in the community, though on a very limited basis—chronic shortages of contraceptives, personnel strikes, and other logistical problems plague the government's system. The former clinic's steps are used by a tire repairman as a raised platform for his small street business. A sugarcane vendor, with a mound of purple cane stalks stacked high in an old wheelbarrow, leans on the building's wall out front, stripping the tough cane coating with his machete and selling what ends up being breakfast or lunch to hungry residents. Women with heavy loads on their heads fill the area as they wait for local transportation to take them to their marketing sites.

The cost of living has nearly quadrupled since the mid-1990s. There is a somber feeling in Cité Soleil these days, made all the worse by the presence of *chimè-s*—paid street thugs who seem to rule the general anarchy that inhabits this community. When I returned to Cité Soleil in 2003, politics still dominated conversations. Turf wars between gangs involved in drugs, vandalism, and efforts to control the community had only accelerated. Crimes against the innocent were said to be part of common everyday life. Several residents said that someone is killed at least once a week. The same familiar phrase I had heard in the 1990s was

echoed again and again: *nou pa gen jistis* (we have no justice). During a visit in
2003, I sat with Michlet, an old friend, who confirmed what I felt: "We still live in
a *zonn sou tansyon* (area with lots of pressures)—people can take only so much.
You know, we are living in a calamity." His friend standing nearby added to the
poignancy of the moment: "It's gotten to the point where just living is simply a
violation of human rights."

How did a once robustly funded USAID development project in Cité Soleil
reach such dysfunctional levels? What explains the chronic inability to provide
decent reproductive health care services to a group of women and men who, in
surveys, say that they do not want to have more children? And, why did residents
there protest the use of family planning so deliberately?

Throughout this work, the political economy of fertility framework has helped
explain the varied forces that keep fertility high in the community of Cité Soleil.
At each level of analysis—from the household to the donor-driven international
health agencies—shifting terrains of power or powerlessness have shaped and
dictated actors' motives and behaviors. In different ways and in different settings,
individual agency is pitted against structural constraint. In the household, for
poor women faced with limited survival options, sexuality becomes the sole (and
often humiliating) way to access economic power. In the clinic, the transformation
of a family-planning promoter and women's health advocate to CDS informant and
spy was rewarded with fine clothing, jewelry, and access to the inner decision-
making chambers of CDS. Within the medical establishment, the once compassionate family planning doctor became medical director and, in the process, was
transformed into a hardened bureaucrat. And in the community, some CDS
health care workers turned to radical political organizing, while others became
members of the villainous paramilitary FRAPH and used their health care skills
to undermine the poor. For both organizers and FRAPH, these transformations
offered increased political status and economic incentives. The CDS general director, formerly an avid public health advocate, by virtue of his class and political
savvy became a political figure central to USAID's activities and the promotion of
their world view. And when CDS collapsed in 1996, even President René Préval, a
seemingly staunch defender of the people's democracy, yielded to political pressure under the threat of losing all health care funds and forced his Ministry of
Health to accept the terms of USAID's health-care plan for Cité Soleil.

These multiple perspectives have helped identify *what* lies behind high fertility and *why* family planning is so problematic: gender, culture, and economic
and political power all come into play. In this chapter, I examine *how* this problematic situation evolved by tracing the history of international involvement in
Haiti from colonialism to the present. Grounding the ethnographies of the households, clinic, and community of Cité Soleil in the larger context of Haiti's history
rounds out this political economy analysis, providing a critical element for

understanding and responding to the cries for health and justice in this community and in this nation at large.

History, McNicoll (1993b) reminds us, is instrumental in the construction and transformation of social institutions, which inform our understanding of fertility change over time. Failure to place contemporary questions about the Haitian population crisis into a historical context has led to an oversimplified diagnosis of Haiti's so-called persistent population problem. By retracing Haiti's history in the first part of this chapter, I explain how a series of historical, political, and economic forces since the time of colonialism have shaped the high fertility and low contraceptive use found in Haiti today. In the second part of the chapter, I focus on the national and international responses to this "crisis" ever since it was first identified as such, by a Haitian demographer, in the late 1950s (Moral 1961). The evolution of what became a U.S.-driven population program in Haiti from the 1970s onward demonstrates how political and economic forces, rooted in postcolonial structures, inform the way that international aid is provided to this beleaguered nation today. From this perspective, it becomes clear how resistance to these structures, echoed in the voices of despair from the households, clinic, and community of Cité Soleil, has played a relevant and persistent role in determining Haiti's demographic destiny from slavery to the present day.

History and Demography: Explaining Population Growth

Slavery and Economic Expansion

Intimately tied to economic expansion throughout Europe and the Americas, Haiti's population growth can be traced back hundreds of years, to the Spanish and then later French colonization of the western half of the island of Hispaniola, then called St. Domingue. By 1789, St. Domingue supplied two-thirds of all overseas trade of goods imported into France and was the largest single market for the European slave trade. At its peak, St. Domingue was considered the greatest colony in the world and called the "Pearl of the Antilles" (James 1989:ix).

By the late 1700s, the population of Haiti was divided into three groups: primarily 40,000 white colonialists, the 30,000 "free" mulattoes (generally children of colonialist men and black slave women, granted nonslave status by their fathers), and approximately 450,000 black slaves, who worked as house servants or field hands and were born in and exported from Africa (Farmer 1988b; Fass 1980; de Saint-Méry 1958). Although there were a substantial number of people inhabiting the island during this early period of slavery, harsh working conditions and resulting ill health inhibited fertility and kept birth rates generally low (Fick 1990). Impatient plantation owners, who needed more labor to expand production, calculated that the cost of importing a slave was considerably less than the cost of supporting a child from birth to adolescence, when he or she could start working. But as the cost of imported slaves increased around the mid-1700s, plantation owners recalculated and took on a decidedly proactive maternal and child health interest (Curtin 1990). Efforts were made to reduce miscarriages and infant mortality among the slaves on the island. Pregnant slaves were given more medical care and time off during the late stages of pregnancy and while nursing. Awards were even given to mothers of several children.

Brodwin's rich review of the history of medicine in Haiti (1996) offers a fascinating view of Haitians' earliest signs of political resistance. Women's reproduction was at the heart of that resistance. Bougerol (cited in Brodwin 1996:42) shows how abortion was a sign of rebellion—or an "attempt to decimate the work force, and hence the owner's profits." Reportedly, torture and confinement were common punishments for abortions. Early on, the reproduction of slaves was determined in large part by plantation owners and colonial powers. In this way, "the regulation of sexual relations," contends Stoler (1991:57) "was central to the development of particular kinds of colonial settlements and to the allocation of economic activity within them."

A second factor triggering significant demographic change came from European and later American economic expansion in Haiti. The period of slavery that spanned almost two hundred years on the island of Hispaniola established a pattern of large families that did not end with slavery. Bloody slave uprisings led to independence from France in 1804. Haitian leaders immediately attempted to restore the plantation economy. The majority of peasants refused, however, and either bought or reconquered land from the state in an effort to control their own production. The existence of a nation-state of former slaves was threatening to the leaders of Europe and North America, particularly those in the American South, where slavery was still common, and so Haiti was soon isolated from the world economic system (Smith 2001).

This, however, did not stop internal profiteers, who instigated a system of taxation that "turned fiscal and marketing systems of the country into mechanisms that would allow [the elites] to siphon off the wealth produced by the peasants" (Trouillot 1995b:124). These gross economic imbalances produced a small but strong elite class, representing 5 percent of the population, composed of property owners, merchants, professionals, and government members. As they do today, Haiti's educated and French-speaking aristocracy lived in the largest cities (primarily Port-au-Prince, Cap-Haïtien, and Jacmel), practiced Catholicism, and maintained a "Western" outlook and behavior in all respects, including marriage followed by domestic family organization (Fass 1980:14). The remaining 95 percent of the population were peasants, rural farmers who spoke only Haitian Creole, were uneducated and illiterate, and tended to have more common-law unions (a legal marital ceremony was too expensive) (Trouillot 1990). Traditionally, birth certificates produced by the state officially classified members of Haiti's lower classes as "peasant."

When the United States finally recognized Haiti as a sovereign country in 1862, economic ties were secured by means of exports of raw materials. Coffee, one of Haiti's main exports, was planted, tended, harvested, processed, and then packed by peasant farmers. Typically, coffee-producing peasants lost up to 40 percent of their income to federal taxes (Farmer 1988b:88). Other exports such as cotton, indigo, rum, cocoa, and mahogany, much of it cultivated on small plots of land, put a premium on large families. As the export-oriented economy demanded produce from an increasingly poor and land-impoverished peasantry, children were needed to increase—or even maintain—household production. Throughout this period, family size remained high to maintain pace with required production (Cordell and Gregory 1987). Thus, structural forces rewarded maximum reproductive performance.

Once the United States staked economic interests in Haiti, political interests soon followed. Decades of political instability plagued Haiti from the mid-1800s and through the first American occupation of 1915. Haitian historian Leyburn is often cited for his apt description of the era: "Of the twenty-two heads of state between 1843 and 1915 only one served out his presidential term in office, three died while serving, one was blown up with his palace, one presumably poisoned, one hacked to pieces by a mob, and one resigned. The other fourteen were deposed by revolution after incumbencies ranging in length from three months to twelve years" (Library of Congress Country Studies, n.d.).

The American occupation of Haiti, sent to bring "stability" to the weakened nation, lasted nineteen years, from 1915 to 1934. Once installed, the United States supervised all governmental decisions in the country, including how best to deliver health care to the nation, the effects of which have been far-reaching. The establishment of a public health care system in Haiti had two significant effects on population change. First, the Americans introduced a highly rationalized and technically driven health care system, thus setting precedent for the equally technically driven family planning programs that define reproductive health care in Haiti today. And, second, the introduction of public health programs affected key demographic indicators—mortality and fertility—but in unexpected ways.

Laying the Groundwork: The Public Health System in Haiti

The nineteen-year tenure of the American occupation, according to Brodwin (1996:48–49), "radically transformed medical institutions and practices in Haiti." By 1919 the country was divided into distinct geographical and bureaucratic regions, and by 1925 there were eleven hospitals, a training school, and sixteen rural dispensaries throughout the nation. Less than five years later the Americans were directing the medical school and sending graduates to the United States for advanced training. Mass inoculation programs for yaws and smallpox followed. Although Haiti's rural population may have been healthier, United States control of the public health sector through the occupation served to lay the groundwork for ongoing power struggles that now define public health, medicine, and the development aid on which Haiti is so dependent today.

Following the occupation, the public health effort directed by the American Sanitary Mission during World War II brought more disease-control campaigns to the country, along with a tightened bureaucracy and highly structured schemes, all followed up with increases in international aid. Increasing access to public health services served to increase rates of population growth, since the introduction of immunizations led to a decrease in childhood mortality, but without the anticipated decrease in fertility that the demographic transition model predicted. Although progress in public health has been painfully slow, and still does not reach millions of landless Haitian peasants, life expectancy increased from age 47 in 1960 to age 56 in 1992 (UNICEF 1994:72) but, according to UNICEF (2003a), life expectancy has recently decreased to 49 years of age.

Many Haitians resented the heavy-handed U.S. approach to the development of the public health care system. Brodwin notes that evaluations of the medical reforms that happened during the occupation are mixed. Some, such as Bellegarde (cited in Brodwin 1996:52), claim that the public health grid laid by the Americans "was one of the most useful institutions organized in the country." Nicholls, on the other hand, criticized medical reforms as "largely guided by the need to make Haiti an attractive country for foreign investment" (cited in Brodwin 1996:52). As we shall see, the rapid pace of two waves of urban migration, based largely on new phases of economic expansion in the 1950s and 1970s, gives credence to Nicholls's interpretation.

Migration and Economic Expansion

The first major migration started in the late 1950s, when the increasing rural population struggled to survive on overused land. Impoverished peasants increasingly relied on permanent and seasonal migration both within Haiti and among Caribbean islands. Peasants leaving rural areas contributed to the emergence in cities of a new *klas popilè* (popular class) or proletariat at the bottom of the social structure (at the time, close to three-quarters of the population of Port-au-Prince). The construction of Cité Simone as a "worker city" in the mid-1950s coincided with this migration. Other migrants left for new employment opportunities, notably sugar cane cutting in Cuba and later the Dominican Republic. During the first wave of migration, the bulk of the migrant labor was male and contributed to the relative independence of women in the management of household life that is common to the Caribbean area (Laguerre 1978). Specifically, the migration of males helped produce a domestic pattern of multiple familial units in different geographical locales (Cordell and Gregory 1987). As men migrated, women became increasingly responsible for both the economic and domestic welfare of their children (Blumber and Garcia, cited in Brydon and Chant 1993). Over time, lack of economic stability, linked to scarcity of land and labor, left women with few survival options—except those tied to reproduction, but usually with new partners. This pattern reinforced the serial monogamy now common throughout Haiti and typical of all the women interviewed in Cité Soleil.

A new phase of migration in the 1970s was triggered by the development of the export-market industrial sector through a pact between USAID, several large bilateral aid agencies, the World Bank, and the Haitian government.[1] For impoverished peasants, this development promised jobs. For the United States, poor Haitian peasants would be a source of cheap labor, with Haiti's comparative advantage of being close to the United States. In fact, the industrial sector in the capital never grew to the size intended, jobs were elusive, and working conditions, as women in Cité Soleil recounted earlier, were at best fairly brutal (see NLC 1993). Sexuality and reproduction took on increased meaning and, literally, value as women's options in the workforce dwindled.

It was during this same period, between the late 1950s through the 1970s, that the developed world grew ever more concerned and fearful about the world's growing population and scarce resources, later termed the "the population bomb." The movement to reduce population growth stemmed in part from the growing environmental concerns by liberals in the United States who concluded that population growth was a major contributor to environmental destruction worldwide. The environmental movement failed to fully analyze the problem, particularly the role of the United States in environmental destruction, notably the notoriously gross consumption of resources that occurs in developed nations and therefore their disproportionate contribution to pollution compared with the much smaller amount of resources consumed by developing nations. This growing fear led to a call by the United States and other developed nations for reducing population growth, which ultimately set the course for family planning interventions not only in Haiti but also worldwide (Green 1993). With overpopulation, dwindling natural resources in the countryside, and growing urban squalor, Haiti needed funds for numerous maternal and child health interventions. But Haiti's previous experiences with U.S. public health interventions, most notably during the occupation, were firmly etched in the minds of Haitian doctors working in public health. Dr. Ary Bordes, a former minister of health and long-time pioneer in Haitian preventive medicine, foresaw the effects that the politics of international funding would have on national population control objectives:

There is an obligation for every country to progressively increase its financial contribution to the [population] programme. In the opening stages, outside funding is understandable. But once a government has included family planning in its plans, whether for health or demographic reasons, it must put aside the necessary funds.

International funding is mixed up with international politics. Its fluctuations are not necessarily linked to national needs. A well-found, well-oiled

nationally funded program, with popular participation, can be less costly
than an external one, with foreign ideas and money. (Bordes 1981a:1)

As we shall see, Bordes's insight into the conflict between national and international family planning goals was borne out in subsequent years.

Pigs and Pills: Haitian versus U.S. Strategies for the Population Crisis

As early as 1960, a representative from the Western Hemisphere Region of the
International Planned Parenthood Federation (the same donor that funded the
Cité Soleil clinic thirty years later) first arrived in Haiti to explore family planning
project options. By 1964, the National Council of Family Planning was initiated,
and Haitian-designed strategies took off. Haitians' approach to public health
incorporated family planning as part of larger primary health care and community-based initiatives. One of Dr. Ary Bordes's first projects in Cul-de-Sac, Haiti,
successfully combined community visits by health care promoters with clinic-
based prevention and treatment for sexually transmitted infections as well as for
other endemic diseases. Literacy activities were also an important cornerstone of
this initial project. Bordes was equally aware of malnutrition and hunger as overriding problems, and worked closely with local agronomists to improve food
production. "Pig fattening" projects to boost livestock sales, and revolving loans
to support small business activities, were central to community organizing. This
approach ensured that people's immediate demands for survival were met. Any
spare cash generated could be spent on needed medical treatments. Condoms
were handed out to—and eagerly accepted by—male agricultural workers at each
community meeting. Working quietly, and on lean funds, Bordes's second project,
which integrated two more villages into the plan, replicated this initial success. By
the end of year two, 40 percent of the adult population in their reproductive years
in the three villages were practicing family planning. Contraceptive prevalence
rates in Haiti have never been recorded at such high levels since. In fact, these
rates were nearly three times higher than the national rates in the mid-1990s and
four times higher than the highest rate of use ever recorded in Cité Soleil (Bordes
and Couture 1978; Ross and Frankenberg 1993).

By contrast, from the late 1960s onward, the U.S. agenda in reproductive
health focused increasingly on funding strictly family planning activities. The U.S.
State Department regularly convened "high level" meetings with USAID to discuss
international population policy (Green 1993). All efforts to investigate or further
social and economic development as part of reproductive health care programs
were eschewed in favor of a contraceptive focus (Szreter 1993). Haiti, close to
Cuba, was perceived by the United States as particularly vulnerable to the threat
of communism. Efforts for integrated development strategies with full community participation were seen as socialist strategies for the redistribution of wealth
and were dropped. Policy planners from the United States were adamant: There

was little time to wait for the effects of development with the population growing out of control. Family planning, it was argued, was an *alternative* to social change (Szreter 1993). By 1967 external funding had completely revamped Haitian-designed public health initiatives. Agendas of international donors, on whom Haitians were already reliant, served as an early source of conflict and an enduring obstacle to effective family planning service provision.

Yet early warnings of a contraceptive-heavy agenda were surfacing. In the early 1970s, Gerald F. Murray, an American anthropologist, completed fieldwork entitled "Culture and Fertility Field Work in Haiti Relevant to Family Planning: Progress Report." Murray (1972:63) looked at empirically recorded economic, demographic, and attitudinal phenomena around the issue of fertility, in a rural village, and concluded: "If one takes a deep and comprehensive look at the situation in rural Haiti, one is forced to conclude that current family size is not an accidental demographic blunder that can be remedied by the diffusion of contraceptive knowledge and practice but rather a systemic component which is geared to the demands of a particular type of economic system. This insight has important implications for family planning programs. *Stated bluntly, it means that the hope of demographic stabilization through contraception is a pre-scientific pipedream*" (emphasis added).[2]

Development experts around the world resorted increasingly to interventionist approaches to help coax fertility down—thereby, it was assumed, speeding up the process of economic development. This approach commenced simultaneously in different regions throughout the world, and by the late 1960s and early 1970s dominated the policies of international population control agencies with mixed results (World Bank 1993a). The top-down, vertical program objectives focused primarily on ensuring full access "to a variety of contraceptive methods; to satisfy unmet need and intention to use a method; to reach the desired fertility level; and to attain the replacement fertility level" (Ross et al. 2000:69). This agenda allowed policy makers in the West to "focus on the supply of family planning services rather than the promotion of economic development and infrastructure projects which in turn might engender demand for birth control" (Szreter 1993:674). Providing contraceptives through "vertical," family planning–focused delivery (rather than integrated development) was a development policy with a clearly technical solution that paved the way for the contraceptive-heavy approach used today.

When Instability Pays Off: The Political Economy of Population Programming

Under pressure from USAID headquarters in Washington, D.C., all official public health endeavors from 1971 onward were to have separate population components. Haitian programs and project activities were reformulated according to USAID protocols and standards. Bordes's projects, in spite of their notable and sustained successes, were refused funding in the early 1970s by both the International Planned Parenthood Federation and the Population Council because they represented a skewed perspective, one that was "for so much more than family planning" (Bordes and Couture 1978:173). Although grants continued to pass through the Ministry of Health, project content was completely determined by international funders (Bordes and Couture 1978).

By the end of the 1970s, it was clear that family planning programs in Haiti were not following the "successful" patterns reportedly emerging in other parts of Latin America and other regions of the world.[3] Foreign observers of Haiti's population strategy claimed that since 1971 the Haitian Ministry of Health had a "virtual monopoly" on family planning activities. In addition, "A lack of commitment to make use of that monopoly . . . has impeded any serious increase in contraceptive prevalence beyond a mere 6 percent of women in union, despite enormous assistance provided in this field to the Government of Haiti by the international donor community" (Guengant and May n.d.:iii). Another international agency corroborated this view: "The Ministry of Health exerted close control on family planning activities; however, given their lack of recognition of the urgency of family planning education and service development provision, this has resulted in a virtual standstill in the development of private nonprofit and for-profit initiatives" (CARE-International 1990:2)

Because of this pervasive distrust of the government bureaucracy as a conduit for family planning funds, during the next decade the U.S. government began an aggressive campaign to privatize health care through private voluntary and nongovernmental organizations. This policy, which is still in effect, has increasingly removed control of family planning from Haitian public health officials.

During an interview with one of the CDS family planning doctors who formerly served as a key population advisor to the Haitian government, the power of U.S. political and economic domination became clear. He explained to me, in explicit terms, how U.S. population assistance in Haiti moved in two well-calculated stages: first, from an integrated to vertical service provision strategy, and second, from a ministry-controlled funding status to private sector control of virtually all family planning funding. "It was a massive blow," he recounted, "leaving the public sector with almost no resources. There was no way to survive. The U.S. had a fundamental change in attitude about the Haitian government after the 29th of November, 1987." This date marked what USAID called the "abortive elections"—Haiti's first effort at democratic elections, scarred by a "savage murderous spree on innocent voters" and orchestrated by the tonton makout-s and the military as part of Haiti's post-Duvalier "hesitant march towards democracy" (USAID 1993).

In reaction to the Election Day massacre, the U.S. government, Haiti's largest aid donor, cancelled approximately 60 million dollars of proposed economic aid for 1988 as well as a small amount of proposed military aid. An additional

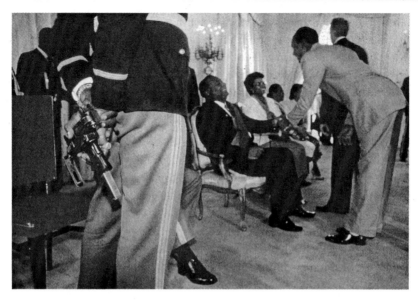

Inside the National Palace: Manigat, one of three heads of state during 1988

34 million dollars of economic assistance, all of it distributed by private voluntary organizations and nongovernmental organizations, was not affected, since it was not channeled through the Haitian government (Inter-American Commission on Human Rights 1988).

International aid was now dependent on Haiti's ability to create a stable "democracy." With each successive government and change of ministry (or restructuring) that has occurred, USAID's decision to work almost exclusively within the private sector, through selected Haitian and American NGOs, had been validated. U.S. policy was responding to the instability and corruption of the Haitian government; the policy further weakened the public health sector by curtailing funds for broader purposes and narrowly targeting family planning goals. "Democratic" conditions, defined by the United States, not Haitians, continue to determine how aid flows to Haiti. Since an electoral dispute in May 2000, the United States has pressured the Inter-American Development Bank to block US$512.9 million in development and humanitarian loans. Of that sum, over 20 percent is targeted for health care services (Shakow 2003).

Evaluations of private sector family planning activities express a chronic "inability" to cooperate with the Haitian government in several different ways.

> The inability of A.I.D. to provide support to the public sector constitutes
> a barrier to project success. In principle, there should be some comple
> mentarity between the public sector and the PVOs [private voluntary
> organizations] involved in health/FP [family planning] service delivery, in

order to affect adequate geographic medical coverage. Simply, some of the MSPP [Ministère de la Santé Publique et de la Population (Ministry of Health and Population)] facilities, which should serve as reference facilities, are barely functioning.

The inability of USAID and other donors to work with the GOH [Government of Haiti] in other sectors constitutes a second barrier in this regard. In theory, population and family planning cannot be isolated from other sectors. Over the last few years, however, the suspension of donor assistance across-the-board—of reforestation programs, of assistance to agricultural production, of the drilling of new wells, etc.—has served to isolate FP personnel and programs in most areas.

Finally the political context of the last few years has not always allowed local organizations to function, or has required that they function on a strictly limited basis, and has at times precluded organized meetings necessary to promoting FP (USAID 1993:17).

Steeped in justifications around Haiti's dysfunctional governments and promoting integrated health care and development "in theory" and "in principle" under more ideal conditions, USAID neatly furthered its own agenda of a vertical family planning program while simultaneously undermining an already weak Ministry of Health, keeping it "barely functioning" in the process.[4]

Another reason for favoring the private sector over the government was the widely acknowledged level of corruption in the national Ministry of Health. Development experts at USAID argue that putting money directly into NGOs reduces overhead, graft, and the tendency for funds never to leave Port-au-Prince. Equally, it does away with the need to renegotiate complex contracts and levels of trust with every coup d'état and change of government. The rapid pace of NGO growth in the reproductive health sector in Haiti has enabled USAID not only to enforce U.S. family planning priorities but also distance itself from the complicated, fragmented, and conflictive reality of Haitian society. "The discourse of international development constitutes itself . . . as an expertise and intelligence that stands completely apart from the country and the people. . . . International development has a special need to overlook this internal involvement in the places and problems it analyzes, and present itself instead as an external intelligence that stands outside the objects it describes" (Mitchell 2002:211).

Imaging itself as what Mitchell calls a "rational consciousness," USAID has effectively privatized the population sector in Haiti, defining the terms and conditions of nearly all of its aid. This control of aid has also determined who gets funding. USAID's extensive support of CDS, as a prominent nonprofit, typified this sort of privatization and patronage. CDS as an organization was well liked by U.S. officials not only because most of its upper-level staff spoke English and trained in the United States, but also because CDS bought into the technocratic family planning intervention model that USAID touted—against the will of the people it served. CDS helped perpetuate U.S.-style development, one that failed to consider the larger social, economic, or political context in which the family planning interventions were applied in Cité Soleil. In this way, USAID could control and maintain its own development ideologies by supporting select nonprofit organizations, ensuring full control over the amount of influence and power of certain groups (CDS) over others (its constituents in Cité Soleil and their community organizations). When the Ministry of Health took over CDS after its collapse in 1996, it, too, unwittingly helped perpetuate and maintain the same development ideology.

"On Our Knees:" Population Politics and Resistance

Placing reproduction within its historical context has helped to explain demographic trends over time by illuminating the political and economic forces that have driven Haiti's fertility and international responses to it. Population programming, both locally in Cité Soleil and nationally within the halls of the ministry, has been met with a great deal of resistance. Bell (2001:5) notes that scholars often define resistance by four criteria: "the action must be collective and organized; it must be principled and selfless; it must have a revolutionary impact; and it must negate the basis of domination." But Bell also argues that these criteria are too narrow to fully embrace how resistance is played out in Haitian culture. Her focus on Haitian women as resisting the margins of power, in often covert and unseen ways, brings to fore the way in which the public transcript fails to acknowledge how Haitians defy the institutions or systems that deny them their rights.

Residents of Cité Soleil, through their acts of resistance and accommodation, demonstrated the ways in which the individual and the body politic relate and constantly negotiate. In the community, they actively protested birth control through campaigns against the clinic and pre-FDA–approved methods like Norplant. Likewise, residents' understanding of how a seemingly benign public health program transformed itself into a political vehicle used to undermine their health rights is a powerful reminder that matters of reproduction are full of contradictions (cf. Gutmann 1996; Paley 2001; Parker et al. 2000).

In the family planning center, providers' weak advocacy for family planning, while mired in elitist class issues, can also be interpreted as yet another layer of resistance to family planning as an ineffective public health intervention. Providers' analyses of family planning's general failure, in light of Haiti's social ills, were explicit. These perspectives reveal the specific subjective consequences, local responses, and human costs of hegemonic public health interventions in people's lives. At the national level, in the halls of the Ministry of Health, Haitian professionals practiced more subtle forms of resistance—generally that of noninvolvement—since, as one physician recounted, overtly challenging this control could bring with it the threat of eliminating funding to other poor and starved public health sectors. These strategies show how "even when abuses of power cannot be confronted directly, they are not necessarily accepted passively" (George 2003:162).

This view was corroborated again later in 1991 (under the first Aristide government) when, at the urging of several Haitian colleagues, I helped prepare a prospectus suggesting increased Ministry of Health involvement in private-sector public health activities. The concept paper suggested subcommittees within the Ministry of Health to oversee projects implemented through USAID to ensure ethical field standards, provide improved service delivery coordination between nongovernmental organizations and public services, and avoid replication of services. The then Minister of Health balked at the idea. A Haitian colleague later explained that even the suggestion of some form of control by Haitians within the ministry would not be well perceived by USAID and could threaten the future of all public programs.

My understanding of the tension that exists between Haitian nationals and the international donor community is rooted in a conversation I had with Madame Déjean, the Cité Soleil family planning center's nurse. Madame Déjean had been a part of the family planning center since its inception in 1983. She was a large and handsome woman. Her linen outfits were always neat, though stressed by her size. She wore her hair pulled back tightly, and she had the habit of regularly checking on her bun with her red-painted fingernails. For over ten years Madame Déjean had complained steadily about two things in the clinic: not having a small refrigerator for colas (and "things like that"), and her low salary. Her requests were never heard; in the end, she brought her own cola in a cooler filled with ice. She would often run ice cubes across her forehead and along the folds in the back of her neck to cool off. She sat, preparing cotton balls for the afternoons' Depo-Provera users, soaking each ball in alcohol and placing them in a stainless steel container. Her opinions about family planning were strong and pointed, informed by her long history of working in this clinic: "They [foreign experts] resist us and we resist them. The Haitian people are strong and we won't always do what the foreigners think we should do. I sometimes think it's in the interest of the foreigners for our situation never to change. Still, they have never sat down with us, there are no round tables, to understand what the real problems are—imagine that! They don't understand our problems and they try to resolve them."

Interviews with Haitian physicians and nurses who worked in the public (government) sector were full of resentment over the manner in which family planning programs were designed. One nurse was adamant: "To separate out family planning has never worked, and will never work in this country. Health in Haiti must be viewed as a global effort; it is rare that we are consulted on such matters." With his finger pointing at me, a physician said, "A family planning center, detached like the U.S. model, makes little sense to Haitian women who value their time. What Haiti needs are multipurpose primary health care centers. Why is this so difficult for the Americans to understand?" All of the Ministry of Health employees interviewed during this study favored integrated health programs, not stand-alone family planning clinics, in addition to increased training for personnel. Although they recognized that political instability creates logistical problems, they did not see this as the main impediment to success.

Poor communication and coordination with the U.S.-funded private sector was a topic of concern that surfaced regularly during interviews. So, too, did the extent to which Haitians remarked on their forced dependence on foreign aid and "all of its trappings." An irate physician, referring to the private sector, said this: "Nothing marches to the same rhythm and until there is collaboration, nothing ever will." Another high-ranking Haitian family planning professional within the ministry, who asked to go unnamed, complained, "Since long ago, we've been obliged to get on our knees in front of USAID—and in our own country! They control all the issues."

As an adaptive mechanism to this imposed control, many members of the Haitian medical community have been determined to avoid this unidimensional family planning approach. For example, the Ministry of Health offers family planning, but almost always within the context of maternal and child health services. Although physicians acknowledged that family planning was generally not a successful part of these services, they were quick to point to a paltry ministry budget, a constant shortage of methods, and lack of infrastructure. "How can we implement anything without a penny?" The U.S. private sector's vertical, technology-driven approach has created enormous conflict and, as one physician noted, "distracts" the public sector from taking steps to enhance service provision. One colleague indicated that, if anything, family planning has a "bad name" because it has been pushed so aggressively by the private sector.

Haiti's resistance, on both the part of the *pèp* (the masses) and the government, to accepting vertical family planning interventions further frames the explanation of why a strong population sector has never really developed. In addition to acknowledging that Haitian officials wanted to integrate family planning activities into programs dealing with other pressing issues (such as, nutrition, immunizations, and so on), demographers from outside of Haiti were forthright about the cultural resistance to U.S.-imposed policies. "Some constituencies in Haiti are still reluctant to embark on a large family planning effort which is sometimes viewed in Haiti as an exogenous, American-imposed policy. On the other hand, some leaders are also tempted to respond to the population pressure by launching policies designed at revitalizing the agricultural sector and/or fostering economic growth, therefore minimizing family planning interventions" (May et al. 1991b:5).

The ensuing conflict of national versus international (largely U.S.) priorities is an unexplored though significant factor contributing to the population "problem" in Haiti. Although joint committees and meetings between USAID and the Haitian Ministry of Health are common, tensions remain strong. A high-end official at USAID's health office summed up U.S. indifference to Haitian involvement in the sector: "There's no one worth anything over there," referring to the ministry employees at the Division of Family Hygiene and Nutrition. Animosity among Haitians toward Americans is equally strong, though few overtly challenge this control. Vertical family planning programs, like those long espoused by the United States government and many of the U.S.-funded agencies, have never had the full support of most Haitians (Bordes and Couture 1978, Bordes 1981a). Global forces have determined the terms of accepting population "assistance" and, according to Haitians, this has compromised (both financially and logistically) nationally devised strategies for more comprehensive health care.

For Haitians, increasing dependence on foreign assistance has translated into an increasing loss of control, and power, over project design and crucial program aspects at almost every stage of the sector's evolution. Surrendering power over the design and control of the family planning sector reflects struggles of power and national sovereignty on a much larger scale. The resistance is not new to Haiti; it is rooted in decades, if not centuries, of protest against external forms of economic, political, and public health control that began with the slave insurrection in 1791 and persists in modern-day Haiti.

Pushing Practice and Policy—Haiti Joins the International Population Arena

Pushing U.S.-style family planning programs in the midst of what is a divisive and damaged national setting has required considerable perseverance. U.S. policy to provide contraceptives—in spite of all the coups d'état—has been a constant since the sector was first funded in the 1970s. In the next section, I show how this practice is rooted in a "rational" model of family planning which assumes that individuals freely choose contraceptive technologies if they are made available. I go on to explain how, in order to support this "rational" approach to service delivery, it was necessary to create an enabling environment in which the model could effectively function. Two separate mechanisms, institution building and policy making, have been used in an attempt to create an environment conducive to the success of the model. This model of service delivery, bolstered by very specific and efficient public health institutions and a policy that recognizes Haiti's "population problem," effectively frames a development agenda that is both technical and antiseptic, removed from the reality of poor people's lives. Here, I review these elements as essential components to Haiti's entry into the international arena of population players—an arena that Haitians have been refusing to enter for forty years.

"The Blueprint": Family Planning and the Rational Model of Behavior

The provision of family planning, as a response to high rates of population growth, has traditionally been designed not only as vertical and technically driven but is also built around rational behavior (Mott and Mott 1985). This essentially microeconomic model of behavior places the rational individual as the central and prime determinant of fertility change. Women and men are perceived as individuals who make informed choices about both contraception and reproduction. The model assumes that high fertility is a health risk and can be controlled with a scientific technology, or contraceptives. It assumes that because the cost (and risks) of having a child and keeping it healthy are generally high, it would naturally be in women's and men's best interests to avoid these costs. The incentive to use family planning, then, is increased so as to avoid the costs of bearing and rearing children in the context of poverty.

A simple supply-and-demand model like that used in the Cité Soleil family-planning center reinforces the expected rational model of behavior where the concept of a consumer with the power of choice makes good, practical sense. The behavioral model requires that family-planning clients be abstract, rational individuals, seeking a technological and distinctly biomedical solution for their unwanted fertility. Such rationality does not tolerate the social, cultural, or political worlds in which clients live.

This rational model of health care delivery is an example of what Ferguson (1994:256) calls the "intentional blueprints" for development practice, producing a highly visible, "technical mission to which no one can object." What development experts have overlooked is that the rationality of those who are absolutely (or relatively) powerless is almost always subordinate to the rationality of the dominant classes. The very terms used to define health care delivery in Haiti make this point clear—social "marketing," contraceptive "commodities," "supply/demand," "preference," and "opportunity." Critics like Sen (1994:64) suggest that this process is indeed geared toward "manipulate[ing] people's choices through offering them only some opportunities (that is, family planning) while denying others, no matter what they would have themselves preferred." These are also "the reigning ideologies in public health that favor efficiency over equity" (Farmer 2003:18). To be optimally efficient, this model has required significant institutional support—institutions that a politically turbulent Haiti could not readily provide. Decades of steady "institutional capacity-building" in Haiti has helped fill that void.

Institutional Capacity-Building

For years one of the USAID buzzwords in Haiti was "institutional capacity-building." Bereft of functioning administrative or political institutions, policy planners from the United States have filled the yawning gap in Haiti with donor funds targeted specifically toward institutional development. The Haitian Community

Health Institute (Institut Haïtien de Santé Communautaire), Haiti's first school of public health, built in Cité Soleil and affiliated with CDS, was one such effort. The school became the national training site for health and family planning promoters as well as for classes and seminars for professionals at all levels. Although the institute has filled an obviously important need and has trained over 14,000 health professionals since 1986, the courses reflect health needs and strategies determined by international donors. Courses are provided for three distinct levels of health care specialists: for doctors and nurses, for auxiliary nurses, and for field workers. These levels reflect (and replicate) the social hierarchy that contributed to troubled encounters in the family planning center.

One of the institute's stated areas of "intervention" is "technical assistance to institutions for the organization, implementation, and follow-up activities for health and family planning," clearly conceiving family planning as separate from the primary health care program (INHSAC n.d.). Family planning promoters from NGOs throughout the country who attended the institute's courses complained that there was a "ceiling" to what they could learn and found the courses redundant year after year. Yet the institute monopolized continuing education, and often only USAID grantees could gain access to courses. All of the training reflects agendas instituted through NGOs funded by USAID; American consultants have designed most of the syllabi. Other efforts geared toward institution building have occurred through the years. For example, USAID provided scholarships for promising young Haitian doctors sent to the United States to earn their masters degrees in public health. When these certified students of public health returned, they were guaranteed higher salaries and promotions, and so became part of the new public health guard in the private sector, one paid for and controlled by the United States.

At the local level in Cité Soleil, the effects of institution building through the private sector's public health initiatives had far-reaching effects, well beyond simply the provision of public health care. Alongside the institutional effect of consolidating CDS power, CDS's work to provide health services also served to depoliticize poverty and silence the "democracy" that people were so intent on reclaiming as theirs. The family planning program and the ancillary public health services in the community became part of what Ferguson calls the "anti-politics" machine. This, says Ferguson (1994:226), is the "fundamental contradiction in the role that 'development agencies' are supposed to play." In an analysis that speaks to family planning efforts as much as any other development initiative, Ferguson continues:

> On the one hand [interventions] are supposed to bring about "social change," sometimes of a dramatic and far-reaching sort. At the same time, they are not supposed to "get involved in politics"—and in fact have a strong de-politicizing function. But any real effort at "social change"

cannot help but have powerful political implications, which a "develop-ment project" is constitutionally unfit to deal with. To do what it is set up to do (bring about socioeconomic transformations), a "development" project must attempt what it is set up to not be able to do (involve itself in political struggles).

Plans constructed to lower fertility and improve the general health of resi-dents in Cité Soleil clearly failed. "But 'failure' does not mean doing nothing; it means doing something else and that something else always has its own logic" (Ferguson 1994:276). When CDS became the center of controversy, and especially when it hit the pages of the *Washington Post*, USAID became part of the problem. This was neither "planned" for nor expected. "Yet, because the discourse of development must present itself as a rational, disinterested intelligence existing outside its object, USAID could not diagnose itself as an integral aspect of the problem" (Mitchell 2002:234).

Nothing seemed to deter the poor as they protested family planning and CDS's symbolic and institutional power. For both USAID and CDS it proved much easier just to close down services in Cité Soleil and eventually hand the fractured system and the fractured community over to the Ministry of Health as a consola-tion prize. This conveniently reinforced USAID's control of the health care sec-tor—and laid responsibility for failure back on the Haitian government. In what is now a common pattern, the government settled for a form of economic and political control that has choked Haiti since her earliest days of colonialism.

At the regional level, "institutional capacity-building" within Haiti has pro-vided the technical assistance, expertise, and management skills that the country is clearly lacking, at least from the perspective of USAID (cf. Mitchell 2002). In Nepal, Adams (1998) has shown how, in strikingly similar ways, the development industry trains medical urban professionals in the very development episte-mologies it promotes. The aggressive promotion of family planning through NGOs (both foreign and Haitian), coupled with the promotion of research and training that reflects U.S. interests, has been a consistent trend in the develop-ment of Haiti's family planning sector. This outcome has served to reinforce U.S. ideologies about how the population problem is defined and how it should be resolved.

While the United States has pushed institution building to serve its own pop-ulation control purposes, Haiti, as a nation, has suffered from general institu-tional decay.[5] Rather than working with the Haitian Ministry of Health to reinforce, supplement, and encourage the ministry to provide quality services while also assuring some level of accountability, USAID has circumvented Haitian institutions altogether. This, in turn, has eroded the state's ability to perform as an "ideological and cultural container" (Trouillot 2001), thus weakening national ideas about how best to solve the population problem or, as the next section shows, how to design a policy that truly translates into on-the-ground practice based on Haiti's reality.

Making Policy: Rhetoric versus Reality

Even making population policy, a task the Haitian government has been slow to tackle, has centered on private-sector support from the United States. The POLICY Project is a nonprofit organization based in Washington, D.C., that "works with host-country governments and civil society groups to achieve a more supportive policy environment for family planning/reproductive health, HIV/AIDS, and maternal health" (POLICY Project n.d.). The organization's goal is to "fill the reproductive health policy void resulting from a severely weakened public sector. The project seeks to strengthen civil society's role, build public-private sector partnerships, and support the public sector's strategic planning process" (POLICY Project n.d.). Working in Haiti, the POLICY Project, in 1998, helped establish a new post, the secretary of State for Population, created under the Ministry of Health. The then-secretary worked hard to produce an "official" population policy. Two years later the policy was presented publicly on International Population Day in July of 2000, although the extent to which the United States (or Haitians, for that matter) views this as "official" policy is questionable.[6]

The policy begins: "This policy is the result of a laborious process of sensitization, of studies, of thought and analyses, in which—at one level or another—different sectors of Haitian society have been involved, including the international community" (SEP 2000:1, my translation from French).

Although it is highly unlikely that the majority sector, Haiti's nearly eight million poor, were involved, the policy does address reproductive rights in a broad and multisectorial way. It acknowledges that the "emphasis" of the policy "was mainly placed on the numerous connections that exist between population and development and on the need to satisfy the needs of each man and each woman, rather than achieving purely demographic objectives" (SEP 2000:2). The policy reflects, in writing, the International Conference on Population and Development's recognition of the need for "harmonization" of social, economic, and demographic priorities within the territory of Haiti. It acknowledges maternal mortality, food security, the environment, reproductive rights, youth, and women as critical components of a functioning national program. Equally, the strategic plan includes the management of demographic variables (maternal and infant mortality, birth and fertility—including HIV and STIs—and migration), the promotion of gender equity, a "plea" in defense of reproductive rights as well as in defense of integrating demographic variables into Haiti's other sectors (education, agriculture, and so on.) for a well-rounded development. Institutional development within the government is seen as key to fully implementing the policy. Family planning, per se, is a very small part of this *politique;* "vertical" programs are never mentioned, and the private sector is mentioned only once and as "partners." Dr. Ary Bordes, now deceased, would have praised this remarkably comprehensive policy that reflects national needs.

The making of a population policy is something that Richey (2002:9), in a review of African reproductive health issues, says is significant. "Signing a national policy is a symbolic statement to the international community that a country recognizes that it has a population 'problem' as defined in a particular way and that it is a candidate for foreign assistance in the realm of family planning programs. While there is still debate over the nature of the population 'problem,' the existence of a population policy suggests that a[n] . . . apparatus with goals of fertility reduction is at work."

The new "landmark population policy," led by USAID, complete with a "Partnership Commission" to promote common ground between public and private sector health experts is, at least in theory—and certainly rhetorically speaking—a major step forward to unite two contentious sectors (SEP 2000). But at the level of implementation where family planning practice occurs, the U.S. bias toward the private sector is clear. A close look at USAID's major family planning subgrants and contracts reveals that they are clearly weighted toward "over 30 PVOs [Private Voluntary Organizations] and Haitian NGOs" (USAID 1999:18). Public health funding is distinctly separated into "three critical health systems: essential drug/contraceptive commodity logistics, HIS/MIS [health information systems/management information systems] and financial management" (USAID 1999:19–20). Not only are the public health sector's duties highly bureaucratic and rational in scope, but there is no mention of improving the public sector's inadequate geographical coverage or of working toward integrating family planning programs that have been isolated from other sectors. Rather, public-sector activities funded for the next five years are designed solely to support private-sector functions while further enforcing efficiency and reproducing inequities.

In interviews, medical professionals in both the private and public sectors recognized Haiti's population "problem," but their solutions to addressing the problem differed considerably. In practice, the U.S. government's insistence on private-sector support of a vertical population program is still not widely accepted by many Haitians, who continue to advocate for a multisectoral public health approach. The making of a rhetorical population policy officially identifies the population problem, but is unlikely to change the unsuccessful course of family planning programs in Haiti if the United States continues to insist on pushing its own form of practice and forcing Haiti back "on her knees."

Perpetuating Inequities: Coups d'Etat and Contraceptives

Haiti's most recent political uprising on February 29, 2004, marked the country's thirty-third coup d'état, once again ousting President Jean Bertrand Aristide. Testimony to the ongoing influence of the United States on Haiti's political landscape, U.S. involvement was overt: "American officials, who provided the plane that took him into him into exile, say Mr. Aristide left willingly to avoid bloodshed. Mr. Aristide has said his departure was a 'modern-day kidnapping'" (Polgreen 2004:1). This most recent coup d'état, which the United States had more than a hand in fomenting, is a blunt reminder of yet unresolved regional power struggles—which pit the hemisphere's poorest country against the world's most powerful.

In a familiar stance, skeptical Haitians viewed the unelected interim government and its foreign backers with suspicion (Polgreen 2004). Gérard Latortue, the named prime minister, also a lawyer, business consultant, and seasoned United Nations career diplomat from southern Florida served to maintain current U.S. ideologies about foreign assistance and Haitian development strategies (Prengaman 2004). Under these circumstances it is doubtful that things will change, and political decisions in Haiti, be it coups d'état or contraceptives, will continue to be made by those peripheral to Haiti's suffering.

At the root of Haiti's instability—made worse by an increasingly sick, impoverished, and politically incensed population—are inequities, themselves embedded in the centuries-long history of slavery, colonialism, occupation, and, more recently, the heavy-handed practice of development in this small island nation. In many ways, the discourse of fertility and family planning that has been deployed by the United States for well over forty years is a vehicle for sustaining many of these inequalities. The PEF framework unravels and exposes the local and global connections, which in Haiti often intersect in conflicting and contradictory ways. In this case study of family-planning practice, these tensions were expressed between women and men in their hot one-room households of Cité Soleil; between clients and doctors in a clinic bereft of care; between political activists and paramilitary killers in the community where human rights violations were commonplace; between development experts and professionals in the halls of the Ministry of Health—or USAID—where policy and practice were at extreme odds; and, finally, even in Haiti's National Palace, where the United States ushered out one government and hand picked another.

On a macro level, political instability and economic degradation in Haiti affect every aspect of life in the country. The perpetuation of poverty is now a predictable pattern: The elites and the international aid institutions that support them continue to ignore the gross social disparities and distress of the poor, and with each political upheaval, Haiti's barely viable infrastructure and tenuous markets are threatened. On a micro level, the poor in Haiti suffer from these structural jolts in increasingly dramatic ways. When the fragile hand-to-mouth economy breaks, so, too, do the livelihoods of the poor who are desperately dependent on their small, daily cash exchanges.

Reproduction (as a survival strategy) and family planning as the proposed intervention are intimately bound up in the process. For Haitian women and men, already constrained by so many unwieldy political, economic, and social institutions, birth control, as offered in Haiti and more specifically in Cité Soleil, was just another restraint imposed upon their lives. This explains, in large part, Desermite's response to my question, first noted in chapter 1, "But why did you stop using family planning?" With clenched fists, and a piercing stare, she crossed her wrists and said: "Because it enslaved me." Testimonies from women and men, as well as Haitian professionals, indicate that family planning alone is not the solution to their social ills. For these reasons, resistance to using family planning is easier than challenging the forces against it—history, culture, gender, economics, and politics. Refusing to use family planning is one way in which people's protests against larger international structures of domination are expressed.

The PEF framework clarifies how both ideologies and structural forces have operated to promote a version of population control that may run counter to what Haitians really want, or more important, need. Without a multilayered analysis, the real and perceived interests of donors and recipients are difficult to explain—or respond to. The power of population ideology, as articulated by the current U.S. government, is employed worldwide. In the next and final section I will show how it is under these conditions that power, and the abuses that it engenders, become transnational in scope (Trouillot 2001; Farmer 2003).

Pushing Further: Policy and Geopolitics

Although Haiti's history with the United States reflects hemispheric struggles over population ideology and practice, recent policy developments suggest how U.S. population ideology now transcends borders. On January 22, 2001, just three days into his administration, President George W. Bush helped the world see how very important ideologies about demography, gender, and development truly are. In a brief memorandum to USAID, Bush, the forty-third president of the United States, imposed the "Global Gag Rule" and immediately changed the fate of hundreds and thousands of people worldwide.

In essence, the Global Gag Rule is, "a throwback to 1984, when President Reagan first imposed the restrictions, which were then revoked by President Clinton in 1993. It uses the power of the purse to control what foreign family planning organizations do and say with their own funds. Under the Global Gag Rule, foreign family planning agencies may not receive U.S. assistance if they provide abortion services, including counseling or referrals on abortion, or lobby to make or keep abortion legal in their own country" (PPFA n.d.).

Under the ruling, providers', not just clients', rights are curtailed. Reproductive health providers cannot discuss the full range of options, including the availability of abortion, with clients facing an unplanned pregnancy. Opponents say the restrictions "defy medical ethics, preventing doctors from fulfilling their

responsibility to provide complete information to their clients. This sort of government intrusion into the doctor-patient relationship would be intolerable in
the U.S.—yet this is exactly what the Global Gag Rule does in other countries"
(PPFA n.d.: 1). In August 2003, the president extended the gag rule beyond USAID
funding to include "family planning grants" awarded by the State Department.
This move serves to impose ideology while "obscuring the fact that U.S. family
planning assistance funds family planning, not abortion. Since 1973, the Foreign
Assistance Act has prohibited the use of U.S. taxpayer funds for any abortion
services abroad" (Center for Health and Gender Equity 2004:1). The effects of this
ruling leave some of the world's poorest countries without any reproductive
health services.[7]

The assaults in what some are calling the "war against women"—and to
which I would add men—have not stopped there (*New York Times* 2003). These
assaults are both nuanced and bold. For example, the current U.S. government is
also controlling the use of language within numerous international agencies,
including the World Health Organization (WHO), the Pan American Health Organization (PAHO), and UNESCO. Recently, notes Germain (2003:5), while drafting a
WHO report, "the U.S. . . . demanded . . . the . . . purge [of] all references to abortion and use of the term 'reproductive health services.'" A year after reinstating
the global gag rule, the Bush administration took steps first temporarily in January 2002, and then ultimately in July 2002, to deny the release of US$34 million
intended for reproductive health programs funded by the United Nations Population Fund (UNFPA). Blocking these funds will further deny thousands of women
worldwide vital family planning services.

The fixation on language again surfaced four months later, in November
2002, when the Bush administration, at the Fifth Asian and Pacific Population
Conference, "threatened to back out of a landmark United Nations (UN) population policy, ratified by 179 nations in 1994 at the Cairo convention, if the terms
'reproductive rights' and 'reproductive health services' were not removed from
the language of the agreement" (Feminist Daily News Wire 2002a:1).[8] According
to the Feminist Daily News Wire (2002b:1), "Bush's decision was made based on
unsubstantiated claims that the UNFPA supports forced abortions in China. Bush
made this decision despite Secretary of State Colin Powell's earlier endorsement
of the UNFPA's 'invaluable work' and a report from the administration's own fact-
finding team found no evidence that the UN organization 'has knowingly supported or participated in the management of a program of coercive abortion or
involuntary sterilization in China.'" As quickly as the United States backed out of
its commitment, the European Union stepped in with US$32 million for the
UNFPA (Geitner 2002). Haiti is among the twenty two countries slated to receive
these funds.

Under public outcry, and following the work of several congressional appropriations committees to reverse this decision, the Bush administration shifted

the denied funds to the jurisdiction of USAID for programs in Afghanistan and Pakistan.[9] From the transnational perspective, the proposed redistribution of the US$34 million to Afghanistan and Pakistan, two countries intimately tied up with the post-9/11 anti-terrorism initiatives, shows just how much public health agendas can collude with both ideology and, ultimately, geopolitical control. Germain (2003:2), describing the "lethal" nature of these policies and their on-the-ground implications for women around the world, makes an important point: "In a word, the Bush administration's unilateral and dominating approach to world affairs is antithetical to democratic processes, including civil society partnerships."

While global in reach, population ideology, politics, and practice can also have very real and profound local impacts. Throughout this book, we have seen how control and power interact with gender, culture, economics, and politics, weaving their way through the levels of the PEF in Haiti. The health programs that USAID financed for CDS exemplify in a significant way how these multiple forms of power, nested in historically rooted ideologies about development and international population assistance, have served over time to further reinforce the antidemocratic structures that Haiti has shouldered for hundreds of years. These same structures also create and perpetuate the conditions that maintain Haitian women's and men's positions in society and subsequently keep birthrates high. These, in the end, are the forces of fertility in Haiti, forces consistently reproducing inequities.

In the next and final chapter I make some preliminary suggestions on how, locally and globally, we can begin to address these forces, even in small ways, as they move toward a much larger goal of reclaiming their most basic health rights.

7

Health in Haiti

Producing Equity

[Since] we don't necessarily have good responses to the root causes of
poverty and social inequality, we have to take on the symptoms at the
same time.

–Paul Farmer, XIV International AIDS Conference, Barcelona

The political economy of fertility (PEF) analysis that I have undertaken at the
regional and national levels has documented the "politicization of aid" (Farmer
2004a: 1485–1486) that has pervaded the long history of health policies and
practices in Haiti. The study of a family planning clinic in a poor Haitian
community has shown, moreover, how praxis-oriented and politically engaged
ethnographic research delineates how and where local and global forces intersect. The same process uncovers the multiple mechanisms that explain why
Haiti's family planning program lags so far behind other programs around the
world. To begin, family planning policy has been tied to a neoliberal political
agenda that is increasingly focused on "free-market orthodoxy and privatization" (Pfeiffer 2002:193). The initial design, developed mainly by U.S. donors, was
an attempt to rationalize and organize health care delivery in a small country
seen as unable to control its burgeoning population. The logic behind the policy has been deceptively convincing: The nation's economic problems are due
to an excessive growth rate; the solution is to reduce the birth rate, so the trick
is to get people to use contraceptives. Haitian government resistance to this
approach from the outset, coupled with decades of political instability, has dissuaded international aid agencies from involving the government in their interventions, funding private sector initiatives instead. Nearly all of these initiatives
require vertical family planning program models that overemphasize fertility
control while neglecting other pressing public health and social issues.

As a result, Haiti's most recent demographic assessment offers little reason
for optimism. The national contraceptive prevalence rate among all Haitian
women is 15.4 percent (EMMUS III 2000), but the supposed associated benefits
of using birth control do not seem to have come about. The total fertility rate,

which has failed to drop for nearly forty years, remains at 4.7 (EMMUS III 2000), and estimates for 2005 are as high as 5.02 (CIA 2005).[1] Maternal mortality rates are still among the highest in the world. According to recent estimates, Haiti is the one country outside of sub-Saharan Africa that has a maternal mortality rate of 1,000 deaths per 100,000 live births (USAID 2002, UNICEF 2003b). The prevalence and risk of acquiring sexually transmitted infections (STIs), including HIV/AIDS, is the highest in this hemisphere, and women's social and economic status remains among the lowest worldwide (EMMUS III 2000; Farmer 2004a; UNICEF 2004). These statistics, as abstracted as they are from women's reality, speak for themselves: More needs to be done.

The case study in Cité Soleil has shown that a significant part of Haiti's "population problem" rests in fact with the health and international aid communities that have failed to specify what the real problem is and for whom it is a problem. Recently donors to and within Haiti have come to surprisingly similar conclusions about the health sector's development. In July 2004, 250 national and international experts representing the Haitian government, the Inter-American Development Bank, the World Bank, the European Economic Commission, and the United Nations, coordinated a process with the aim of charting Haiti's future course within what the group calls an "Interim Cooperation Framework (ICF)." Their analysis is frank:

> The donors recognize a lack of coordination, of consistency, and of strategic vision in their interventions. These donors have often set up parallel project implementation structures that weakened the State, without, however, giving it the means to coordinate this external aid and to improve national absorptive and execution capacities. . . .
>
> It is important to note . . . a mutual mistrust between the private and public sectors and a lack of partnership between these two entities, particularly in the area of productive investments. Beginning with this transition period, it must fall to the State to set priorities and to play the role of regulator in order to optimize the effectiveness and consistency of external assistance. (Inter-American Development Bank et al. 2004:26)

These calls for an effective, functional, and harmonious ministry of health and international agency partnerships are worthy but, certainly as things stand, unrealistic, given the absence of constitutional rule in Haiti. The reality today, reflected in a recent report announcing the development world's newest measure—the Failed States Index—ranks Haiti tenth most at-risk for state collapse worldwide and describes the nation as "about to go over the brink." (Foreign Policy and the Fund for Peace 2005:1; Fund for Peace 2005). When Haiti experienced its thirty-third coup d'état in February 2004, long-held political and class conflicts devolved into national anarchy. In Cité Soleil, schools and hospitals are closed, nearly all aid organizations have left, the police station is empty, and the

UN peacekeeping forces rarely enter the community. According to a *New York Times* reporter, the political vacuum left in this newest post–coup d'état era has served mainly to "stoke the flames of gang violence. [Haiti is now a place] where everyone knows someone who has been killed recently" (Kamber 2004).

To restore some semblance of a health care system to Haiti, it seems obvious that both a legitimate elected government with more enlightened policies and robust financing for health care are needed, and these changes must be intimately tied to an entirely new logic of large-scale international aid. I have shown in this PEF study how the forces of high fertility involve complicated configurations of history, gender, culture, economics, and ultimately politics. The political aspect of the analysis has focused on inequities inherent in the flow of aid from the rich north to the poor south and highlights the disparities in stakeholders' perceptions of the problem and their commitment to solutions within this very complex development situation.

This chapter considers the practical implications of the political economy of fertility analysis that I have undertaken. It is divided into three sections. The first seeks to answer several crucial questions that arise from a political economy analysis. Is it at all useful to study an internationally sponsored family planning program (or similar health interventions) in Haiti (or elsewhere) using this approach? Does the political economy approach to fertility lend itself to solving the vast problems it describes? What does it mean to bring diverse and marginalized voices into the public sphere, especially if these voices make the logic of development aid less easily understood and even more controversial? The second section narrows the focus to Haiti by reviewing information about four reproductive health programs there that have met with some success. The final section, based on the PEF analysis and this review, examines the most critical question of all: What interventions in fact work.

Practice and a Political Economy of Fertility Analysis

My use of the political economy of fertility framework in Haiti is closely aligned with work in critical medical anthropology (CMA) that also "emphasizes the importance of political and economic forces, including the exercise of power, in shaping health, disease, illness experience, and health care" (Singer and Baer 1995:5).[2] Early writings on CMA and the political economy approach, true to their Marx-Gramsci-socialist traditions, were about political perspective and philosophy (Singer 1986; Morgan 1987). Solutions, usually implied, were expected in terms of popular (or activist) response when people understood their true state and the forces that created it—that is, through consciousness raising within poor communities (personal communication, Fass 2004). Often these perspectives did not lend themselves easily to clear identification of direct action. This disconnection between thought-analysis and practice-action surfaced as a topic of debate within medical anthropology when critics of CMA claimed that the then-emerging field was long on words but short on application (Johnson, cited in Singer 2003).

As a result, critical medical anthropologists soon turned to the issue of application beyond the academy. Singer (1995), building on Gorz's notion of "nonreformist reform," urged anthropologists to unmask rather than mystify the sources of social inequality and ill health. Today, many of the field's leading scholars are as much activists as they are academics (Baer et al. 1997; Singer and Castro 2004; Farmer et al. 1997; Kim et al. 2000). This activism comes with an inherent risk "in a world that (in various and sometimes quite painful ways) punishes those who call reigning structures, groups, and practices into question" (Singer 2003:1). And yet this risk has not deterred political economy (PE) and CMA researchers from undertaking and advocating major changes in numerous health-related areas: tobacco use (Nichter and Cartwright 1991; Stebbins 2001), infectious diseases (Farmer 1997; Ward et al. 2004), syringe exchange (Stopka et al. 2003); organ trafficking (Scheper-Hughes 2002), and primary health care (Paley 2001), to name only a few. In the area of reproductive health as well, PE/CMA scholars have advanced the field by analyzing reproductive health inequalities in health care practice (Inhorn and Van Balen 2002; Richey 1999b; Doyal 1995), HIV/AIDS prevention programs (Campbell 2003), family planning policy and practice (Castro 2004; Kaler 2004a, 2004b; Qadeer and Visvanathan 2004), reproductive health practitioners (Davis-Floyd 2004, Towghi 2004), and the social marketing of contraceptives (Pfeiffer 2004a). In applying their research to practice, these researchers align themselves as advocates of the people whom they are studying while effectively engaging their research "subjects" as able agents of change.

Still, medical anthropologists using PE/CMA approaches have produced only a small body of local ethnographies that directly examine the effects of foreign aid and NGO activity. This book adds to that literature by specifically examining the "interface between expatriate foreign health agency workers in the field, their national counterparts, and the poor communities they are supposed to serve" (Pfeiffer 2004b) in the context of family planning. The practical results of these kinds of analyses are, I think, two. In the field of public health it works to shift predominant understandings away from those generated by biomedical, demographic, and epidemiological research. The latter paradigms remain far too removed and abstracted from the social environments that effect health and well-being. Rather than a static portrayal of a fertility rate that refuses to budge and a nation averse to modern methods of contraception, for example, my analysis explains the dynamic resistance to family planning on every level of Haitian society; how few choices people have when they can actually access health care; and ultimately what risks are taken when either providing or using contraception. Here, the PE/CMA approach is particularly useful in that it exposes the complexities behind birth control too often portrayed as a simple public health solution in many poor communities, whether inner-city Pittsburgh or downtown Port-au-Prince, where women are said to be having too many babies or men too much sex.

Second, the PE/CMA investigator may make direct interventions while in the field. As a "barefoot ethnographer" (to borrow Scheper-Hughes's term again), I was deeply engaged in the lives of the women and men of Cité Soleil, turning my data, collected in as objective manner as possible, into real-world applications. Collective organizing in Cité Soleil, in spite of political instability, became a natural vehicle for promoting the local health care reforms, no matter how small. For example, during the research period, working with the family planning promoters and several of the more prominent grassroots organizations, we collectively addressed three important family planning issues: clinic staffing, client education, and the appropriateness of certain contraceptive methods.

Poor doctor-client issues (highlighted in chapter 4) and strained community relations (covered in chapter 5) were partially addressed by creating the position of family planning promoter as part of the formal clinic staffing structure. The promoters, many of whom were nonliterate, were trained in both literacy and reproductive health. Their positions generated employment, helped them access public health education, and promoted what we had hoped would be improved quality of care outside of the clinic in the community and homes of potential and actual clients. Often promoters would help women confront issues around gender inequalities in their homes, holding conversations that were impossible in the clinic setting. The family planning promoters of Cité Soleil were among the nation's first lay reproductive health experts, and they successfully trained scores of promoters around the country.

A second achievement of the engaged PEF approach, also produced with the family planning promoters, was the collective design and publishing of educational materials targeted for low-literacy audiences. These materials served to educate women and men about method choice as well as potential side effects. The materials successfully countered the clinic policy of not informing women of potential side effects.

Third, based on clients' concerns and complaints, the promoters worked with community groups to question the appropriateness of the Norplant method. Together they challenged the use of this method in such a resource-deficient setting, where the clinic was unable to help clients cope with the method's particularly difficult side effects. Ultimately, questions about the manner in which the Norplant acceptability trial was carried out brought to light improper method-removal practices, which were acknowledged by health officials only much later and led to improved training and new national standards of care.

Although these changes may seem small in light of all the things wrong with the clinic and delivery of services, they were positive accomplishments for the poor of Cité Soleil. Through the process of studying family planning with the eye of a critical medical anthropologist and by virtue of the engaged stance taken, we were able to test the feasibility of different strategies—and in most cases improve services. However, we rarely had full institutional support. For example, to their credit, CDS supported the design, pretesting, and publication of educational materials, created by a Cité Soleil artist. The materials, used during national training seminars, were popular in almost every corner of Haiti; they were informative, funny, and explicit. However, a staff member who worked in the Health, Population, and Nutrition office of USAID deemed the materials "obscene" and ordered them banned. CDS complied. Although the materials never won full support within Haiti's international health agencies, promoters and grassroots groups made sure that they were widely dispersed through national underground networks. Years later a new USAID population officer, perhaps lacking institutional memory, remarked on how "creative" and "positive" they were. Many of the concepts, illustrations, and images were then copied and used in USAID-funded reproductive health educational brochures for years afterward.

Applied systematically at the local level, where critical anthropologists do their work, a PE/CMA approach could accumulate in a body of research about action solutions, not just problems. As Simon Fass, an economist and long-time scholar of Haiti, astutely remarked: "One would then have the stuff not only of hegemonizing processes, but also de-hegemonizing processes" (personal communication 2005). Although a PE/CMA analysis may not solve the vast problems it describes, especially at the structural level, it often highlights areas where smaller, more targeted interventions can "take on the symptoms" of inequality, one natural step at a time.

Reproductive Health Results: Quiet, Small, and Powerful

Given Haiti's position as a nearly "failed" state and what I have portrayed generally as a "failed" reproductive health care sector and specifically a "failed" family planning program in Cité Soleil, an important question remains: Can poor Haitian women achieve better reproductive health care short of somehow escaping poverty?

In the final two sections of this book, I focus on reproductive health programs that have had some success in confronting many of the forces of fertility in Haiti. The review focuses on four different programs developed over that past twenty years that are situated in very distinct communities: two in urban locales—one within an industrial park zone, another in a slum community—and two in rural areas. Rather than suggest reforms, I focus on results. Highlighting what has made these programs work is a first step toward revealing some of the de-hegemonizing processes around reproductive rights that are already under way in Haiti.

Center for the Promotion of Women Workers

Wedged next to the main industrial park in Port-au-Prince is the Center for the Promotion of Women Workers (CPFO, its French acronym), founded in November 1985 through an initiative of the U.S. government. CPFO initially offered programs focused on workers' rights, including a training program to educate Haitian women about their legal rights as factory workers. This program included information on the Haitian political process, human development, literacy in Haitian Creole, and broad reproductive health education, covering women's general health, family planning, HIV/AIDS, and first aid. Women who were sexually abused or coerced on the factory floor were given access to a lawyer on staff at CPFO, who works closely with two local feminist organizations also addressing women's rights writ large.

As a result of advocacy by women workers, CPFO opened a clinic in 1989, focusing on family planning provision, prenatal care, gynecological exams, and dermatology services. The single goal is to provide in a comfortable, private setting quality care that also educates women about how to take charge of their health. Clients are invited to attend a monthly course in sexual health provided by one of the female CPFO physicians. In addition to the program's clinic services, CPFO has an extensive field program and sends "motivators" to the state-run industrial park (SONAPI) where workers of both sexes are educated about HIV/AIDS, STIs, and gender. CPFO publishes the *Jounal Fanm Ouvriyez* (Working Women's Journal) ten times annually, and this information is provided to clients during factory training sessions. Most of the journal's content is written by women workers themselves, especially the members of the Komite Ouvriyez pou Defann Dwa Fanm nan Faktori (Committee of Women Workers to Defend Women Workers' Rights, or KODDFF, its Haitian Creole acronym). The work of KODDFF, an urban-based popular organization that meets monthly, is to discuss working conditions in the factories, how these conditions affect women's lives in their neighborhoods, and strategies to reduce all forms of structural, local, and physical violence against women. CPFO, in partnership with women workers in the area, commemorates several international health and workers' days such as the Women's Day, Health Day, Labor Day, Literacy Day, the Day of Protest against Violence against Women, and AIDS Day. More recently, CPFO has organized a successful HIV/AIDS peer educator program where citizens who have been trained in HIV/AIDS and other STI prevention strategies spread information throughout their home communities by raising awareness of infectious diseases, distributing condoms, and referring potential clients to CPFO services. Peer educators also occasionally participate in educational forums, sometimes held on the factory floor. The success of this integrated service approach is reflected in CPFO's comparatively high contraceptive prevalence rate of 38 percent at the end of the first quarter in 2005—23 percent higher than the national average (personal communication, Djénane Ledan 2005).

Association for the Promotion of Comprehensive Family Health

The Association for the Promotion of Comprehensive Family Health (APROSIFA, its French acronym) is based in Kafou Fèy, a poor, very densely populated

Port-au-Prince neighborhood with characteristics similar to Cité Soleil: high unemployment, disenfranchised citizens, persistent egregious levels of crime, and environmental conditions that make survival difficult.[3] Health and sanitation in this zone are among the worst in the country. Housing, often perched precariously on rock cliffs surrounding the main road, is crowded with extended families and other dependents who have fled from rural poverty. APROSIFA's mission since its inception in 1993 has been to promote the well-being of the family, with its focus on women living in the zone. Initially, the clinic provided comprehensive maternal and child health services, including ob/gyn care, internal medicine for adults, vaccinations, laboratory testing, infectious disease treatment, information and education on sexually transmitted diseases, psychological services (for women suffering from rape and/or spontaneous abortion), and finally, family planning. In its second year the clinic's activities were expanded to include an active AIDS prevention campaign, launched with extensive outreach activities (songs, dances, concerts, theater productions, and more). The campaign served to raise levels of awareness about the connectedness of reproductive health to other aspects of people's lives.

Twelve years later the clinic has further expanded and now provides, in addition to a nutritional center for mothers and babies, literacy classes for mothers, and mothers' clubs that address issues of social justice and women's rights. The program translated and published the first Creole edition of *Where Women Can Find No Doctor* (Hesperian 2004) and subsequently designed a national training program around effective community use of the book. APROSIFA also now includes a popular sexuality and health program for adolescents and a small crafts project that generates income for HIV-positive women. Regular outreach services in the areas of education, clinical and medical care follow-up, and family planning promotion (including distribution of condoms) make up the community services. All of these activities are coordinated by a mixed group of community organizers, administrators, and clinicians.

Improvement in health care access for residents in the heart of this rough urban community is remarkable. Family planning services have increased annually. APROSIFA's contraceptive prevalence rate in 2003 was 24 percent, 9 percent higher than the national average (APROSIFA 2003). APROSIFA's main obstacle today is depleted contraceptive stocks that the Ministry of Health has been unable to fill. From 1997 to 2002, nearly 98,000 people received integrated reproductive health services. During that same period, over 25,000 were reached through educational activities and referrals to the clinic.

Deslandes Community Health Center, Albert Schweitzer Hospital

The Hôpital Albert Schweitzer (HAS), is based in Deschapelles and was founded by physician Larry Mellon and his wife and partner Gwen in 1956. HAS provides comprehensive services, both preventive and curative, to nearly half a million

Haitians living within a 610-square-mile area of the Artibonite River Valley. Though the hospital has weathered and continues to confront political and administrative problems, the women's health program, nested within the Community Health Department, has been remarkably effective.

As part of an effort to provide improved services to women of all ages, the HAS/Women's Health Program (WHP) began in 1999 with intensive planning activities followed by service implementation in the year 2000. The Women's Health Program's strategy embraced an integrated package of reproductive health services to women of reproductive age (15–44 years of age) while also enhancing services to adolescents and men in need. Client contact is made at the household level and includes the dissemination of health education for family planning, prenatal care, good nutrition, and infant and child health care. The Deslandes Community Health Center, one of fourteen different health centers served by HAS, is in an extremely remote mountainous town, with roads impassable during the rainy season. Deslandes's isolation makes it an ideal site for the pilot Emergency Obstetric Care (EOC) project, designed to address high rates of maternal mortality in Haiti. Based in a small room at the Deslandes dispensary, the EOC project's equipment is remarkably simple: one table, one bed, and a minimal amount of required medical supplies. Births are attended to by one of three auxiliaries who received training at HAS; nurses attend births when available. An impressive system of referrals has also been established in order to ensure that patients are sent to the main HAS/Deschapelles hospital if a mother's or baby's life is at risk. This is no small feat in rural Haiti. When a transfer occurs, the Deslandes nurse radios village assistants who carry the patient on a stretcher over two kilometers to the river's edge. There, the patient is transferred to a dugout canoe to cross the river and then carried another kilometer to the main road. A vehicle from HAS eventually meets the patient, who is almost always accompanied by the village midwife as a patient advocate. In order to raise awareness of the need for rapid transportation in cases of obstetric complications, the project is widely promoted among schools, churches, youth clubs, community leaders, and health committees.

Preliminary results of the pilot project have been encouraging. Since its implementation in February 2004, the project helped thirty-three women and assisted with seventeen births. That is thirty-three Haitian mothers' lives potentially saved. The relatively low number of births is indicative of the project's design as an emergency alternative to local midwifery care. Midwives continue to play a critical role in the program; because of their training in identifying complications during late stages of the pregnancy or just prior to birth, they typically bring high-risk patients to the EOC program in Deslandes. Midwives are an important community resource, and HAS does not wish to replace or duplicate their services. Notably, and based on the comprehensive and supportive reproductive care and education provided to all women, adolescents, and men in the community, contraceptive prevalence rates in Deslandes for 2004 were 30 percent, double that of the national average. HAS is currently incorporating STI diagnosis and treatment as part of its standard reproductive health service.

Partners in Health

In another rural setting, deep in Haiti's Central Plateau, is Zanmi Lasanté (ZL, a Partners in Health affiliate), a private, nonprofit community development organization founded in 1988. From the start, ZL staff knew that poverty and gender inequality were cofactors in most diseases that strike Haitian women. In 1990, ZL founded its Women's Health Project, which provides prenatal and postnatal care, vaccinations for women and children, and screening and treatment of sexually transmitted infections and cervical cancer to women who had no other source of health care available to them. Women's "agents," trained in all aspects of reproductive health education, serve as critical links to many of the very remote villages covered by ZL services. When lack of condom use or faithfulness of male partners proved to be problematic to women's overall health, ZL produced several innovative prevention models, culturally relevant videos, and theatrical performances. Many of these HIV/AIDS information and education programs proved to be equally effective among Haitians in Roxbury, Massachusetts, as they were among peasants living in the Central Plateau. Prevention videos depicting life stories of people living with HIV/AIDS were regularly shown on national television. Since then, ZL has developed four strategies for HIV prevention and care within public health clinics, all of which overlap with basic reproductive health care. Consequently, during primary health care visits at the clinic, physicians encourage HIV prevention in the following four treatment areas: HIV prevention and care including voluntary counseling and testing; tuberculosis detection and treatment through directly observed therapy; women's health and family planning; and diagnosis and treatment of all STIs.

In 2001, the women's health clinic expanded to a women's health center building at ZL to provide prenatal, obstetric, and gynecological care throughout their widening catchment area. By 2004, over 4,000 women had been tested for gonorrhea and chlamydia. Women are also tested for HIV, syphilis, and trichomonas. This aggressive approach to STI diagnosis allows ZL to provide timely treatment of sexually transmitted infections and to coordinate testing and counseling for HIV with prevention education and condom distribution. In 2004, the program screened 3,500 women for a variety of infections and conducted hundreds of interviews in an ongoing effort to build a database of case-control information in rural Haiti. In 2004, ZL was well above the national average of 15 percent for contraceptive prevalence among its poor rural constituents and plans to train nearly 240 new women's health agents to be supervised by nurse-midwives in their rural villages (personal communication, Loune Viaud 2005; Walton et al. 2004). Over time women are being treated for a host of reproductive diseases that normally go unrecognized and untreated in Haiti. Treating these diseases is an essential first step in a successful public health prevention effort that includes family planning.

Far from being submerged by a wave of international goals and resolutions or swept aside by a barrage of numbers and targets, all four of these programs have been quietly delivering results to the communities they serve. Their programs provide unique reproductive health strategies designed for their particular local populations. This is not to say that these programs have fully succeeded in giving all women at risk for pregnancy a viable family planning option, but in the end they are providing comprehensive health care and working toward feasible goals of equity and access in the communities where they work. When these basic goals are achieved, then family planning will finally become a real choice.

What Works? A Case for Comprehensive Reproductive Health Care

This study of family planning in Haiti reinforces the important message that reproductive health is a complicated and regionally specific phenomenon, rooted in local as well as global economies, deepening poverty, migration, gender, and cultural politics. Although piecemeal solutions through public or private efforts such as those of CPFO, APROSIFA, HAS, and ZL are unlikely to change Haiti's demographic outcomes, these small, focused projects point to effective models of responsible health care that respond to local needs—even in the midst of national turmoil. Testing the success of these interventions can easily be accomplished by comparing the effects in another group without the intervention. Individual donors can be held more accountable, especially when goals are modest. Developing feasible health care models like these, combined with further critical ethnographic research that attends to understanding the social and health impacts of these activities in situ, is important. In spite of all the factors that have sent Haiti down its deteriorating path, Haiti's poor can, I believe, achieve a better level of reproductive health care.

The dearth of decent reproductive health care is certainly a pressing need in Haiti. But the bottom line remains: Poor Haitians need far more control over the entire health care process. In the final section of this book, drawing on what works—and what doesn't—I propose four essential conditions for providing basic reproductive health care in Haiti: an integrated, coordinated system of care; diversified and flexible funding sources; full community participation; and accountability.

Coordinated Care

Whether or not health services should be "integrated" (also referred to as "horizontal") as opposed to "vertical" has long been debated in public health circles.

Integrated services are those that are part of a larger health care and community service delivery system, while vertical services are those strictly earmarked for a particular intervention. The merits of vertical versus integrated approaches in public health, as I argued in the previous chapter, are context and program-dependent. In Haiti today, the vertical approach has been successful when addressing TB eradication efforts and HIV treatment programs; studies have shown that vertical programs work best when treatment and prevention are disease-focused (Farmer 2003; Desvarieux et al. 2001).

The vertical, biomedical family planning model used in Cité Soleil, however, was not a viable solution. High fertility is not a disease. Throughout this book, in the household, community, clinic, and the government, people have cogently argued that a focus on high fertility, to the exclusion of other pressing public health issues, ignores the context in which high fertility thrives. Researching the acceptability of family planning in Haiti over thirty years ago, Ballweg et al. (1974) concluded that combining high-quality contraceptives and childbirth care would likely lead to increased family planning use. Prenatal and postnatal care—in the home or in the clinic, depending on the client's health status—ensures continuity of care for clients. Trained midwives throughout Haiti can and want to ensure this type of care. Providing birthing kits to midwives and instructions in the use of scissors, thread, and antiseptic is simple and costs little. With proper preparation and coordination of prenatal visits, births can be planned for in the most appropriate setting: the hospital, outside of the clinic, or in the home, depending on client needs. The Deslandes Emergency Obstetric Care program at HAS makes this point very clear. Creating a referral system between clinics and hospitals for complicated deliveries saves lives and would probably enhance residents' experiences with the entire reproductive health process. Once a healthy birth is completed, the introduction of follow-up care for the mother—including birth control—is a natural step in the health care process.

APROSIFA was the first integrated health center in its zone, and the clinic director is adamant that the clinic's integrated approach has increased the number of family planning clients. Not only was the clinic able to attract clients who were reluctant to seek out exclusive contraceptive services but the clinic's integrated approach also provides support to the strong community-based distribution components of the program. In addition to family planning as one part of basic medical care, CPFO, APROSIFA, HAS, and ZL all also provide education on tuberculosis and HIV/AIDS and counseling services within the same clinic. Three of the programs also provide nutritional support, and two provide housing and educational assistance, financial assistance to generate future income, as well as employment opportunities. When services address more of the risk factors for poverty and health problems, then they are more likely to succeed.

ZL's program from the start focused on reproductive health care, linking contraception to the life cycle from preconception to postconception care. ZL pushed the concept and practice of integration even further. In 2004, ZL joined with Fonkoze/Haiti, Haiti's largest microfinance institution, to address both health and economic issues. Fonkoze/USA, an American nonprofit, recruits individual and socially responsible institutional investors in the United States and Europe to provide foreign capital made of long-term debt and equity. Residents in Boucan Carré, a community of 10,000, are now the beneficiaries of both a new bank and a new hospital, established with the help of the Haitian Ministry of Health. Months later, the partnership expanded to a second community on the Central Plateau of Haiti. Supporting an integrated model of microfinance, education, and health care services, Fonkoze provides microloans, savings, currency exchange, and money transfers to people living below the poverty line, using a solidarity group savings methodology.[4] Currently, it is testing new methods of reaching the very poorest families, especially those living with HIV/AIDS and/or tuberculosis. In addition, Fonkoze designed a progressive course that combines the teaching of literacy with sexual and reproductive health. The primary objective of the program is to change the extent and nature of communication between partners, spouses, parents and children, family members, and friends. The materials involve learners in problem-solving activities, in practicing conversations, in role playing, and in discussing issues having to do with domestic and sexual violence, migration, partner notification, infidelity, peer pressure, and the special risks faced by women living in extreme poverty.

Health care accompanied by social change is not a new model—in places like Kerala, India (Halstead, Walsh, and Warren 1985; Nag 1989), Cuba (de Brun and Elling 1987), Sri Lanka (World Bank 1998), and Costa Rica (Food First, n.d.) notable fertility declines have occurred without an intensive family planning effort. In most of these societies, income distribution is less skewed than in many other countries. In all of these countries, common commitments include income and land distribution, employment and educational opportunities, mass education, improvements in women's position in society, as well as accessible health care and family planning services. And all of these elements have been key concomitants of the decline in fertility (Kabeer 1994:205). All four of the Haitian programs noted in this chapter are working toward some, if not all, of these larger goals.

Finally, all four programs reviewed have put gender equity at the center of their reproductive health goals. For women, especially poor women under the strain of single-headed households, psychological needs are vast. Each of the programs reviewed offers access to psychological services around violence, rape, HIV/AIDS, and other stigma-related issues when developing appropriate treatment and care plans. Throughout Haiti, men are too often left out of conversations around reproductive health. In Cité Soleil men acknowledged that they are key to both reproduction and the spread of sexually transmitted infections. Yet when female clients returned home with a handful of condoms, men often reacted violently. Conversely, many men expressed a genuine desire to be active participants in health care as one way of fulfilling their role as partner/provider. Almost all the men I interviewed expressed interest in having services designed specifically around their needs (rather than as part of the women's clinic). Addressing these disconnections to men is critical to both health and gender equity. A study in thirteen countries, in diverse regions in the world, used men as community-based distributors of condoms and showed very promising results (Population Council 2002). CPFO has integrated some male HIV/AIDS educators onto their team and offers services for men in their clinic. HAS has many men visiting its clinics, especially for STI testing and condoms. APROSIFA's model for male clients squarely addresses these needs through an extensive gender-based educational curriculum and an entire clinic devoted to men for the diagnosis and treatment of STIs. ZL follows a similar model. Both APROSIFA and ZL have partner notification systems so that treatment is as thorough as possible. Incorporating services that address men's sexuality, responsibility, and health needs is an absolute prerequisite for improved reproductive health outcomes.

Funding

In the same way that all four programs have managed to provide integrated care, their funding strategies have been equally innovative and selective. Each of the programs highlighted have focused less on U.S. government funds and primarily on long-term private and progressive donors from the United States and Europe. Two of the four programs are seeking some USAID funding in the future, based on very specific program needs, but such funds are generally overly restrictive. The current U.S. focus on advocacy rather than direct reproductive health service provision does not meet the urgent needs of the communities served by these model programs. Further, U.S. government funds are ensnared in U.S.-Haitian political relationships, which have been contentious at best. Because of frequent political instability U.S. funds are sent to Haiti irregularly, which can, for example, lead to a dangerous interruption in services for clients dependent on monthly or trimonthly doses of contraceptives. Diversified funding sources are therefore mandatory for providing integrated services.

CPFO and APROSIFA have generally relied on several European donors whose agendas reflect broader health care service delivery goals. Careful selection of funding partners has ensured that these clinics can provide services that meet local needs rather than donor-driven priorities. APROSIFA's clinic director notes that all of their current funders "are very open to listening, negotiating, and taking time to understand the orientation of our services." APROSIFA receives aid from European agencies, such as Christian Aid/United Kingdom and Ireland, which recognizes poverty as a major source of the HIV/AIDS epidemic. Oxfam/Great Britain also provides APROSIFA funds for work with teens and youth, including the distribution of condoms in a responsible way. Similarly one of CPFO's funders is Cortaid, a Netherlands-based funding agency that values the integrated approach of CPFO's exemplary HIV/AIDS program and works closely with the needs of CPFO.

In order to sidestep the vertical family planning approach tied to USAID funds, both APROSIFA and ZL relied for nearly a decade on Planned Parenthood Federation of America–International (PPFA-I) funding. PPFA-I relies on private foundations and individual donations as its funding base and, although focused on contraceptive provision in Haiti, its definition of reproductive health is broad and focuses on sex education and gender equity. Instead of demanding vertical programs, PPFA-I grantees in Haiti have been able to broaden their service-delivery approaches.[5] ZL has also relied on private funds from the Open Society Institute for its now well-developed women's health program. Although HAS maintains good relations with the U.S. Embassy and USAID, the innovative Women's Health project, funded by the Gates Foundation, was the single largest grant in the HAS organization's forty-four-year history. The grant allowed HAS to build an integrated service strategy emphasizing community involvement but with high-quality back-up hospital care. In addition, HAS administrative foresight ensured that the five-year grant be stretched to cover services for a sixth year by merging grant resources that addressed related maternal and child health services. Although the Gates Foundation cut funding in 2005 (Haiti is no longer a "priority" country), the HAS Women's Health Program is well poised to attract new funders. Both ZL and HAS have also benefited from sharing joint activities with the Global Fund to Fight AIDS, Malaria, and Tuberculosis and have used these funds to provide education on reproductive health priorities. Diversifying funds and creatively merging similar project activities and goals has helped all of these programs to maintain a solid and mutually reinforcing funding base over the long term.

Although none of these programs is yet entirely self-sufficient economically, they are effectively challenging narrow family planning approaches that do not meet the reproductive health needs of their constituents. The success of these approaches is clear. By addressing fertility and related reproductive health diseases—and, in some cases, issues such as literacy and poverty—these programs are building long-term community health sustainability in cost-effective ways.

The Community

Many of the difficulties in the clinic encounter in Cité Soleil stemmed from the fact that the clients' world was so different from that of the more elite auxiliaries, nurses, and doctors. CPFO, APROSIFA, HAS, and ZL have minimized these differences in two ways: first, by building strong outreach efforts, and second, by addressing clients' needs beyond the purely biomedical realm.

Although it is doubtful that any of these programs have managed to thoroughly break class barriers between health care providers and the general populace in Haiti, in all four programs clinic staff are recognized for their critical work. Nurses generally run the HAS rural clinics, and in Deslandes, a program I evaluated in 2003 and 2005 for the Gates Foundation, the quality of care was exceptionally high. All of the outreach teams of the four highlighted programs provide comprehensive education and medical follow-up. In each program, outreach workers—whether women health workers, health assistants, or community health workers—also take an integrated approach, addressing multiple issues rather than simply refilling supplies of contraceptives, recruiting clients, or providing education limited to family planning. Outreach workers, almost always from the same class and circumstances of the clients they serve, ensure that the clients' first encounter with the health care system is usually with a trusted community member, who also serves as a patient advocate. Community health workers or women's health workers at ZL, for example, are responsible for the assessment of patients' homes in order to determine if there are any risk factors present that could affect either the patients' or community's health. During daily home visits, community health workers assess family members, community members, living conditions, financial status, and nutrition of the family. Within the APROSIFA and HAS structures, women's health workers or health agents work hand-in-hand with peer educators to bring a host of services to clients' homes, including sexuality education, information, referrals, and contraceptive services. At CPFO, outreach workers go onto the factory floor and are largely responsible for recruiting women to the clinic and providing powerful education to help women leverage inequalities both in the home and workplace. Trainers also teach women first aid techniques that they have brought back to their communities. Their presence in and of itself within the industrial park, especially during lunchtime seminars, is a powerful reminder to factory owners, floor managers, and others that poor women have access to their rights.

Relying on dedicated and qualified nurses, community health workers, and other lay health specialists may be the answer to this missing infrastructure that most experts claim is Haiti's greatest deficiency. Full community participation also assures that priorities are set locally, usually by health care personnel and the people they serve, not by demographers and family planning consultants visiting Haiti. In addition to basing services on people's realities, all of these programs' community-based structures have been tested and have survived repeated episodes of political violence without major service disruption.

Because CDS clinic personnel were ineffective, by and large, in helping clients prevent, detect, or treat adverse effects of family planning methods, many women took their quest for therapy elsewhere. This use of multiple "therapeutic options" is well documented in the ethnographic literature on Haiti (Brodwin 1996). Over 90 percent of the community sample visited local healers for a variety of ailments. Healers in Cité Soleil claimed that most of their women clients either sought treatment for side effects from contraceptive methods (bleeding, headaches, and fatigue, for example) or came in search of forms of birth control because side effects of prescribed methods proved intolerable. In Haiti, "teas of leaves and roots represent an inexhaustible base of resources" and are often used in conjunction with pharmaceutical products (author's translation, Bordes 1981b). Doktè fèy-s (leaf doctors), who prescribe traditional forms of herbal medicine, welcomed the idea of working in the clinic, though they doubted that biomedical doctors would ever approve of such a plan. Houngan-s—male vodou priests who are often sought for social and spiritual healing—also expressed interest in helping women and men deal with more social and gender-related issues.[6] Machann fèy-s (market women who specialize in leaves), who offer plants for sale, could provide workshops addressing reproductive health remedies for clients. Indigenous healers, who generally charge on a fee-for-service basis, would benefit by simply establishing a referral system from the clinic. One challenge would be helping biomedically trained staff to understand the broader importance of this treatment option for women. Another could be establishing the efficacy of the remedies; however, Haitian women have long relied on a variety of herbs for reproductive ailments and symptoms, as well as for blood-related problems (Colon 1976; LaGuerre 1978).

Traditional healers in Haiti serve not only clients' clinical needs but also their spiritual needs, and often assist with moral issues. All of the healers interviewed noted that clients using family planning were often seeking treatment for social discord within relationships. When I probed for details, it was clear that the community's indigenous healers' work centered squarely on issues of gender inequity within couples. To improve the reproductive health experience, traditional healers could be included in training and program development, focusing on reproductive health ailments. CPFO and HAS, while not directly working with local healers, hold them in respect. APROSIFA sponsors seminars with indigenous healers as part of its complementary and alternative medicine initiative. And ZL works closely with indigenous healers in all the communities that they serve, and considers healers to be powerful conduits to good health. Inviting traditional healers into the reproductive health care process would be a bold and progressive step signifying to clients that all of their needs—clinical and social—are recognized as important and central to care (Brodwin 1996; Rouzier 1998).

Accountability and Action

I once met with the CDS general director in his office and brought with me a long list of requests from Cité Soleil's residents, replete with ideas on how to reform the community's health care system. It was my understanding that as an NGO, CDS, like the hundreds of other Haitian and foreign NGOs in Haiti, was supposed to play a key role in contributing to the development of the marginalized poor, especially in areas like health care, where the Haitian state lacked both the resources and means. The general director listened patiently, as I recited my list, folded his hands together, leaned toward me, and said, "Your work is good. There's just one problem: you're too close to the poor. You shouldn't listen so much; you'll never solve their problems."

As it turns out, I continued to listen and in the years that followed realized how critical both public action and institutional accountability are to garnering health equity. In the midst of Haiti's nascent democracy, racked as it has been by ongoing economic crisis and repressive regimes, nearly every single demand that came from Cité Soleil's health activists was silenced. Without established mechanisms for accountability to the community, CDS was unable to establish its legitimacy there. This critically interpretive local ethnography of Cité Soleil shows that underneath the large-scale government and development policies, alarming indices, and largely ineffective development practices, there is a cultural logic and alternative rationality that governs health care decision making. As much as residents fought for their health rights as one means of expressing this logic, their gains were negligible. Requests for equal and broad local representation in community affairs went unanswered by the CDS administration. Seasoned community health care workers employed by CDS quit in frustration, shut out of conversations and denied forums for voicing their concerns. Rejecting family planning services—or throwing stones at Tipper Gore's motorcade— became the only means of protesting unacceptable practices by the agency.

Moving from a framework where clients are passive beneficiaries and consumers to active participants in their health care is a critical element for program

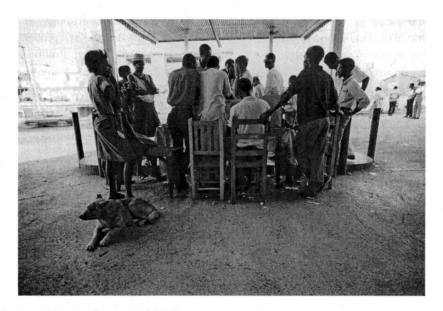

Organizing for change, Cité Soleil

success. CPFO, APROSIFA, HAS, and ZL acknowledge this as central to all their activities. In all these settings—among factory workers or the unemployed urban youth or subsistence farmers in the Artibonite Valley and Central Plateau—local residents sit on health committees and share a voice within the institutions providing services. In some cases, representatives in the community periodically meet with health personnel to ensure that community concerns are heard and that quality-of-care improvements are incorporated into the clinic protocol. Studying the effects of community involvement, Gebrian (1993), working in southwestern Haiti, found that greater participation in "health committees" was predictive of greater acceptance and use of health programs. Democratic organizing, through neighborhood committees, popular organizations, and within small community groups, has a long and rich history in Haiti (cf. Smith 2001). From the late 1980s and early 1990s, residents of Cité Soleil demonstrated, in the midst of ongoing political instability, a remarkable ability to build broad support for democratic ideals and social change. Capitalizing on this fundamental Haitian structure—as part of health care, not in opposition to it—helps explain what works and why.

Accountability moves in several directions. Especially in places of gross inequalities, institutions must be accountable to their clients. Institutionalizing access to health care decision making (about matters such as clinic hours, services, and types of methods offered, and so on) and ensuring that residents are represented and involved would help clinics design more appropriate services that meet the articulated needs of the community. In addition, discussing the community's health statistics, instead of hiding them, as the family planning center typically did, gives residents a greater sense of participation and ownership in the health care system. Shrouding health statistics, the research process, and reasons for intervention-based decisions leads only to distrust. Failure to inform residents about their rights as participants in research also tainted the Cité Soleil community's view of science and the U.S. universities that support it, and yet these studies are important for understanding disease patterns so that appropriate treatment and public health interventions can be designed. A group of U.S. researchers working in Cité Soleil found that "cultural feasibility studies" to "investigate scientific as well as ethical, behavioral, and social issues in the design of clinical trials" are critical in view of the complexity of research designs and the high potential for misunderstood research (Coreil et al. 1998). Partners in Health epidemiologists and clinicians from Boston, along with ZL project staff who understand community dynamics, are overseeing a cluster of studies on the transmission dynamics of STIs in rural Haiti and developing models for flexible application in poor communities worldwide. Research must attend to qualitative as well as quantitative understandings of health and disease.

Equally important, institutions need to be accountable to donors, too. Without a chain of accountability, CDS also failed to openly engage in constructive problem solving with USAID. This stance, typical throughout the NGO community, serves to perpetuate ineffective service delivery strategies. Clinic reports were generated but never used to elicit feedback or comments—except perhaps to blame the promoters for not recruiting clients. Without feedback, what didn't work was funded year after year.

Alternative funding mechanisms with full accountability exist and need to be promoted, tested, and improved. The Global Fund to Fight AIDS, Malaria, and Tuberculosis is one funding mechanism that promotes more accountable, transparent, and participatory development practices. Transparency is reinforced in countries that receive funding from the Global Fund through a country coordinating mechanism (CCM), a national decision-making body with membership from governments and civil society alike. Members of the CCM are from international institutions and national governments, foundations, NGOs and other local organizations, specifically including groups formed by and for people living with HIV/AIDS. Fund administrators insist that civil society members, particularly those living with HIV/AIDS, have a voice. The NGO delegations and HIV+ persons, for example, go beyond simple consultation and are involved in actual decision making nationally through CCMs, and are equal voting members of the fund's board. CCM members send out calls for proposals, decide on national programs, determine funding streams, and ensure follow up, implementation, and evaluation. Once funded, organizations used to delivering vertical health care are encouraged to use horizontal, integrated strategies when appropriate. The Global Fund has no in-country officers or field staff, thereby streamlining costs, while recipient funds are managed, monitored, and also fiscally evaluated through locally contracted financial organizations. This country-focused mechanism also facilitates ownership of the program at the national level. Although still young and on an extremely fast learning curve, being highly visible, with only four years of experience on the ground, the Global Fund is already a significant worldwide undertaking with $8–10 billion spent annually. Undoubtedly the process will be complicated, and there are varying levels of success at the national level, but moving toward a "not-just-business-as-usual" model of equal participation inclusive of all sectors is a substantial step toward leveling the health care and international development playing fields (personal communication, Mark Schuller 2005).

Grassroots participation in the health care process, in and of itself, will not solve Haiti's health problems. If local participation in Haiti is ever to reap positive health outcomes then local attempts by the organized poor must be both supported and enabled by more powerful constituencies—locally, nationally, and internationally. Within communities like Cité Soleil, stakeholders made up of clinicians, clients, and other constituents should agree on mutual and realistic program goals. Donors can then monitor progress, an exercise that if handled ethically and in a fully participatory way can provide an opportunity for constituents to reflect on successes, failures, and needed program changes. Reproductive health donors must shift their axis of thinking around what defines success, especially in countries where fertility decreases have been slow. Although measuring reproductive health outcomes—numbers of clients, methods used, or pregnancies averted—is acceptable, the focus on individual behavior must change. Funding community-initiated activities around health-enhancing sexual norms or safe pregnancies, for example, may be a better long-term investment as an avenue to accepting and accessing family planning than a billboard advertising Microgynon (and written in French). The success of the programs highlighted in this chapter shows that a reproductive health model—with the community as the locus of change—has been critical.

Donors and their powerful constituencies must respond to local needs. The current "advocacy" focus with an emphasis on adolescents (which provides advice rather than contraceptive service provision for anyone at risk of becoming pregnant or causing pregnancy), promoted by the current Bush administration, has pulled needed resources away from basic family planning and reproductive health needs and into narrowly conceived HIV/AIDS behavior prevention programs. In addition to recently shifting the bulk of U.S. money away from the Global Fund to Fight AIDS, Tuberculosis and Malaria, "Bush is using AIDS funds to place religi[ous doctrine] over science, promoting abstinence and monogamy over more effective measures such as condoms and sex education. Before overseas groups can receive US funding, for example, the Bush administration requires them to take a 'loyalty oath' to condemn prostitution—a provision that AIDS workers say further stigmatizes a population in need of HIV education and treatment" (Sealy 2005:1). As I have tried to show in this book, abstinence or monogamy—as part of HIV/AIDS prevention or family planning—in the context of poverty, and where sexual transactions often define the life of an entire household, has little meaning. Strings tied to international aid, especially when driven by ideology serve to reproduce inequities and, can destroy programs, communities, and in the end the people they are supposed to serve. This, in part, is the tragic story of health care in Cité Soleil.

Making the connections—from coups d'état to contraceptives—is essential if we are to understand more fully the ways to make health interventions both appropriate and effective in response to individuals' complex reproductive lives. Revealing the social dynamics of a family planning health care intervention, especially one that has gone unquestioned for nearly forty years in Haiti, has not been a simple or straightforward process—but it is one I am grateful to have participated in.

On my last visit to Cité Soleil in 2004, it was hot and dry, and the sun beat down relentlessly. Within thirty minutes of entering the community, I witnessed two drug deals. There was intermittent shooting from various neighborhoods where I used to socialize, work, and sleep. Several gang members aggressively approached, asking who I was, what I wanted, and an extremely frail man in rags chased after me then hung on my arm pleading for money and medications. Everyone looked defeated or angry. Ernst, a former CDS health worker whom I had known for two decades, hugged me and held my hands as we said our goodbyes. As I got in my rental car, his parting question lifted my mood: "Kati, will you send us your book when it is done?" I beamed back: "Of course!" As we pulled out of the community, I felt determined to finish this work, this book.

When I glanced into my rear-view mirror, squinting in the sun, I saw Ernst again, running from behind the car, smiling and waving his hands. I stopped and rolled down the window and he said, "I forgot to ask! Do you think you could send a dictionary with the book? I can't read English." That will and that desire to learn, to understand and to change the status quo, from deep in the dusty, hot corridors of Cité Soleil is, for me, emblematic of critical medical anthropology and human agency at work even in one of the hemisphere's most calamitous communities. The challenge is to acknowledge fully the multiple forces influencing Haiti's health and fertility and to address reproductive rights as part of a much larger struggle for human rights.

Epilogue

The morgue's ventilation system did not work in April of 2005, when I visited the University of Haiti's General Hospital in Port-au-Prince. The head nurse of the maternity ward and I both covered our noses with handkerchiefs to help keep from inhaling the cloying stench of decaying bodies. The hospital, one of the only remaining sources of health care for the poor of Cité Soleil, has been plagued by intermittent strikes and violence for over a year. The hospital staff fears attending work because, as the nurse told me, "We are experiencing a total breakdown of society." Conservative estimates are that four armed kidnappings of middle-class Haitians, journalists, Haitian businessmen, foreign aid workers, and diplomats occur daily. Just getting to work is dangerous. The poor, too, are at grave risk from random shootings and robberies, and feel unsafe to venture outside, even during the day. Once again, women and girls are bearing the brunt of the brutality, with violent rapes at an epidemic high (MSF 2005). Armed gangs act with impunity as they carjack, kidnap, rape, torture, and hold victims for ransom—and sometimes execute them (Sneider 2005).

Toward the end of my 2005 visit, I had two things left to accomplish: a three-day board meeting with my Haitian colleagues who work with the Lambi Fund of Haiti (a small, nonprofit organization that I cofounded with numerous human rights workers in 1993), and a visit with friends from Cité Soleil. On my way to the board meeting in a small rental car jammed with luggage and laughter from a long-anticipated reunion with committed colleagues, my life and perspective changed precipitously. Our vehicle, speeding along Route Nationale #1, was suddenly surrounded by four gunmen. I documented what ensued—our male driver thrown from the car; three female colleagues and myself kidnapped; guns cocked; a heated, angry dispute about how to rape and execute us—and where to leave our bodies, before they let us run for our lives (Maternowska 2005).

As a colleague poignantly said in a consoling e-mail after the event, "It is one thing to understand people's desperation in Haiti and quite another thing to be its victim." Most difficult to comprehend was that I felt that I knew the men who committed the crime. I didn't in fact know them personally, but they were just like men I had interviewed—and befriended—in Cité Soleil. Accepting the idea that the gunmen who might have raped or killed me might, under other circumstances, have risked their own lives to save mine has been profoundly difficult. At the end of this traumatic experience, I have grasped the fact that the people I care so much about as victims can also be victimizers. Having watched these men grow up under regimes of terror, I know all too well why and how these ugly human transformations take place.

This event brought home, in a very personal way, how terribly debilitating Haiti's political instability is for everyone who works, lives, or simply tries to survive there. Recent developments in Haiti, fueled by centuries-long divisions of class, politics, geography, and national sovereignty, reveal how much the suggestions that I proposed in chapter 7 are only superficial health-policy solutions for what are clearly very deeply rooted structural problems. Simply put, miserable political and economic conditions make it nearly impossible to sustain public health gains. In the midst of the current protracted chaos, international aid has just about ceased, with the result that the already weak public health system has become further destabilized and is now nearly defunct. In addition to devastating national staffing shortages, patients in some institutions have allegedly been assaulted, and hospitals no longer have the basic necessities to

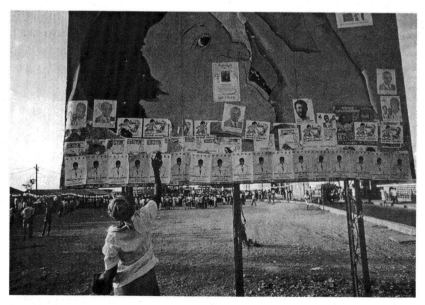

Breastfeeding promotion with political posters, Cité Soleil

function. "It is increasingly difficult to supply hospitals with drugs, medical surgical consumables, water, propane gas, and diesel. Stocks of drugs are not renewed . . ." (PAHO 2004:1). The head nurse confirmed this problem as systemic when she told me that there have been no contraceptives in stock—even in the country's main hospital—for over a year. When I visited a row of fifteen small boutique pharmacies just outside the state hospital, where women and men in need are sent to purchase contraceptives, twelve of them had no contraceptive materials in stock. In two of the three remaining pharmacies, the choice was limited to Depo-Provera, which additionally requires purchasing a syringe and is therefore prohibitively expensive. Haiti's feeble family planning program is, at best, suspended. And the coups d'état keep happening.

The fact that in 2005—after forty years of population control programs—there are nowhere near enough contraceptives in Haiti to influence its birth rate reinforces Paul Farmer's call for an end to the politicization of aid, a practice which "stands as one of the most shameful chapters in international health" (Farmer 2004a: 1485–1486). By launching, adopting, and implementing half-baked, cookie-cutter measures designed to appease one political interest or another, the international community and Haitians themselves consign Haiti to failure. Rather than solve problems, problems are compounded; citizens deserving empowerment are disempowered. People and politicians talk about what Farmer has called the "uses of Haiti," but very few push hard for primary education or basic health care for all. Until that viewpoint is aired and truly infuses the policies and programs of Haitians and internationals alike, Haiti will remain poor and "underdeveloped."

Referring to Haitians during the time of their revolt from France, the historian C.L.R. James has said: "No one had previously conceived that so much power was hidden in a people" (1989: 356). Recognizing this and allowing Haiti to utilize that power once more, on terms defined by and for her people, will be central to Haiti's future course.

APPENDIX

ORGANIZATIONS SUPPORTING COMPREHENSIVE
REPRODUCTIVE HEALTH AND ECONOMIC EMPOWERMENT

CPFO (Centre de Promotion des Femmes Ouvrières / Center for the Promotion of Women Workers). Long established, CPFO provides comprehensive reproductive health care, dermatology, and mental health services to women and men who work or live near Port-au-Prince's main industrial zone. CPFO also works with a legal team to protect the rights of women on the factory floor and in society at large. Contact: cpfo@hainet.net.

APROSIFA (Association pour la Promotion de la Santé Intégrale de la Famille / Association for the Promotion of Comprehensive Family Health). Based in Carrefour Feuilles, Port-au-Prince, APROSIFA manages clinical and social action programs including comprehensive care for adults (internal medicine, reproductive health, and numerous subspecialties) as well as adolescents and pediatrics. APROSIFA promotes health care access, treatment, prevention, and education as unequivocal rights for all Haitians. Contact: aprosifa@direcway.com.

HAS/Women's Health Project (Hôpital Albert Schweitzer / Women's Health Program). Situated in the Artibonite Valley, the Women's Health Project offers Haitian women living in remote rural villages access to comprehensive reproductive health care. Committed nurses, many of whom live and work on the clinic premises, ensure that women receive full emergency obstetric care as well as comprehensive family planning options and treatment for sexually transmitted diseases. Contact: www.hashaiti.org (specify the Women's Health Program).

ZL/PSF (Zanmi Lasante/Pwoje Sante Fanm / Partners in Health/Women's Health Project). The women's health center building at Zanmi Lasante was completed in 2001 to provide prenatal, obstetric, and gynecological care throughout the ZL catchment rapidly expanding throughout the Haiti's Central Plateau. ZL/PSF, based in social justice and addressing inequities that plague Haiti's poorest, offers health care access, treatment, prevention, and education focusing on gender inequalities. Contact: www.pih.org.

SOFA (Solidarite Fanm Ayisyen / Haitian Women in Solidarity). SOFA brings together urban and rural Haitian women to defend their political, economic, and social rights. It supports women's advancement through national policy advocacy, as well as through tangible, grassroots-based projects that make concrete and immediate improvements in the daily lives of poor women; SOFA also offers comprehensive reproductive health care for poor, marginalized women. Contact: lisedejean@yahoo.com.

Fonkoze (Fondasyon Kole Zepòl / The Shoulder to Shoulder Foundation). Haiti's alternative bank for the organized poor is a microfinance institution offering a full range of financial services to the rural-based poor in Haiti. Fonkoze's mission is to build economic foundations for democracy in Haiti. Contact: www.fonkoze.org.

Lambi Fund of Haiti (Fon Lanbi Ayiti). The Lambi Fund's mission is to assist the popular, democratic movement in Haiti. Its goal is to help strengthen civil society as a necessary foundation of democracy and development. The fund channels financial and other resources to community-based organizations that promote the social and economic empowerment of the Haitian people. Contact: www.lambifund.org.

NOTES

CHAPTER 1. INTRODUCTION: WHEN PIGS FEASTED AND PEOPLE STARVED

1. Modern methods of contraceptives offered included combined low dose pills and progesterone-only pills, IUDs, condoms, spermicides, Depo-Provera (injectables offering three-month protection), Norplant (subdermal implants giving five-year protection), and sterilization procedures, by referral to nearby clinics.

2. There is no recent census data available on this community, although one was allegedly conducted, though never finished, in 1993. Several small samples have been culled (cf. Banque Mondiale 1979; de Zalduondo 1991; Godard 1985; Lacombe 1977; Olibrice 1979), and estimates used here are based on these publications. The last known census, completed in the mid-1980s, estimated the population to be approximately 175,000 (Lerebours and Canez 1992). On the basis of a very conservative estimate in 1993 of 180,000 total, approximately 16 percent of the population was women between the reproductive ages of 15 and 45 years and therefore at "risk" of pregnancy (personal correspondence, Despagne 1993). At least 30 percent of the population at that time was less than 15 years old.

3. Six years later, per capita income had decreased to $250, less than one-tenth the Latin American average (Ferguson 1999).

4. It is difficult to determine how credible this estimate may be, given difficult field conditions. However, the research agency collecting the information, the Child Health Institute, is considered by most to be reliable.

5. "Formal" here is defined by the application of the research protocol including, but not limited to, a survey design, sampling procedures, interview schedules, and other elements of the research strategy. Informal data collection, which contributed to the depth of knowledge incorporated in this study, began in 1985 when I first volunteered in Cité Soleil.

6. Following these trips, I participated in press conferences sponsored by the Haitian Refugee Center of Miami. After one, I received an anonymous phone call: "How many times have I told you not to get involved politics?" followed by a disconnection.

7. A report entitled *Haiti-Consular Information Sheet,* dated December 28, 2001, said this about Cité Soleil: "Certain high-crime zones should be avoided when possible. . . . Due to high crime, Embassy employees are prohibited from entering Cité Soleil and La Saline and their surrounding environs. . . . Under no circumstances should anyone attempt to photograph in these areas, as this almost inevitably provokes a violent reaction."

8. By 2003, the gourde had devalued even further to Hg 44 = US$1.00.

CHAPTER 2.   INTERPRETATIONS OF REPRODUCTION: DEMOGRAPHY,
ANTHROPOLOGY, AND THE POLITICAL ECONOMY OF FERTILITY

1. A fertility rate measures the average number of live children a woman has during her lifetime.

2. Fertility rates are usually calculated from crude birth rate measures that are a combination of recorded births and recorded abortions. I can attest that garnering valid birth and pregnancy histories is extremely difficult, especially given the social stigma attached to abortions. Hence, I would argue that the total fertility rate, at least in Port-au-Prince, is probably much higher than the national average, based on information collected during the research and subsequent reports on the prevalence of abortion (TAG 2001).

3. According to USAID in 1991, per capita population activities were $0.83 in Haiti, the highest in the Latin America/Caribbean region, compared to $0.23 in Bolivia, $0.14 in Colombia, $0.27 in the Dominican Republic, $0.29 in Ecuador, $0.33 in El Salvador, $0.47 in Jamaica, $0.16 in Mexico, and $0.31 in Peru (USAID 1991).

4. For example, at the time, contraceptive prevalence was 56 percent in the Dominican Republic, 55 percent in Jamaica, 59 percent in Peru, 30 percent in Bolivia, 41 percent in Honduras, and 47 percent in El Salvador (UNICEF 1994:76; UNFPA 1994:2).

5. Also sharing this dubious distinction are Ethiopia, Angola, Chad, Mali, Niger, Democratic Republic of Congo, Sierra Leone, and Lesotho; all of these countries have had family planning programs with very limited success.

6. When calculating contraceptive prevalence rates, the difference between 6 percent and 10 percent, for example, is not very significant, and it is an extraordinarily tiny trend, if not a zero trend, when one allows for survey response and sampling error.

7. In the year 2000, contraceptive prevalence was said to have nearly doubled to 22 percent. However, during a visit to the capital in 2003, a well-regarded Haitian physician who works in the population sector said this: "These must be false statistics—I have seen evidence of this nowhere." A high-level population representative of the United Nations Population Fund of Haitian origin (whose anonymity I am respecting) agreed with the comment that a stagnant fertility rate—still at 4.7—is also an indication that little has actually changed.

8. In the mid-1990s, USAID managed the entire Private Sector Family Planning Project, an act authorized and initiated in 1987. IPPF and the Pan-American Health Organization (PAHO) oversaw service delivery of approximately thirty-three private voluntary organizations in Haiti. IPPF was directly responsible for the Cité Soleil family planning center. The work of the Population Council focused primarily on developing and testing strategies to improve availability and quality of services within several family planning projects countrywide.

9. In a fascinating review of demography's "science-policy nexus," Presser (1997) traces the history of demography and policy, citing the Indianapolis Study in 1941 as the first national fertility survey. This survey was then followed by a series of large-scale surveys measuring the incidence of unwanted fertility.

10. Carter (2001:166) notes, "Classic structural-functional anthropology decisively rejected its own diffusionist past and with it all versions of diffusion based on simple initiation or contagion." Rather, Carter explains that although elements may move across cultural borders, they are "systematically reinvented in the process."

11. In a personal communication with McNicoll (1995), I presented my point about power. McNicoll responded by saying this: "While that [power] is part of social reality—and in some settings may be a very considerable part—it is certainly not the whole. Accepting such a view would lead into a class analysis, and to portraying that axis of social structure and differentiation. There are . . . other sources of conflict and change . . . in most societies social control works more subtly and in a more multifaceted fashion. Its effects may be barely realized not only by those who are trammeled (hence the consciousness raising agenda of reformers) but also by many of those who ("objectively") appear most to benefit from the situation." I still argue that power plays a crucial and very explicit role in this particular analysis of reproduction and that, in Haiti, social control is rarely subtle.

12. Thanks to Beverly Bell for translating this statement, released in 1986 and one month after the people of Haiti succeeded in overthrowing the thirty-year Duvalier dictatorship.

13. In July 2002, the European Union took steps toward filling the gap left by the U.S. decision to stop funding the UN's family planning organization with $32 million of aid for sexual and reproductive health work in twenty-two countries. This followed an announcement that President George Bush was ending payments to the UNFPA and International Planned Parenthood Federation (Black 2002).

CHAPTER 3.   GENDER AND SURVIVAL: LIVING ON THE EDGE IN CITÉ SOLEIL

1. The areas of motherhood, fatherhood, and parental obligations are only mentioned here as significant concepts that define types of unions and entry into adulthood. Readers interested in this should refer to the authors cited, particularly Lowenthal (1987) for a much more thorough investigation of these culturally defined obligations.

2. The state is supposed to provide free education to children, but the required textbooks or uniforms are prohibitively expensive. There is also a constant shortage of teachers, since most teachers are not paid for the services rendered. Schoolrooms are usually very ragged, with only one room, poor lighting, and several grades present.

3. Fatton (2002) suggests that seven years later, unemployment is now as high as 80 percent nationally.

4. Over one week in January 2003, low-octane gasoline prices increased 75 percent. At the time, Haitian government officials defended the decision to halt fuel subsidies as sound fiscal policy for the impoverished Caribbean country, and refused to cede to pressure. The strike, as well as a series of other economic hardships, has been blamed, in part, on the $80 million national deficit—and on the suspension of hundreds of millions of dollars in foreign aid after disputed 2000 legislative elections (Norton 2003).

5. Sobo (1993), working in rural Jamaica, found an equally difficult situation, where a desperate economic crisis created a context in which living up to the ideals of unions was impossible. Women aimed for stable economic support through sex and childbearing, but they could not depend on the fathers of their children for any support.

6. Handwerker (1993) argues that gender relations structure this violent behavior. Armed with data from three Caribbean countries, the author provides convincing evidence to link family violence, sexual abuse, and level of sexual activity as a generational phenomenon.

7. Industrialists, elite landowners, and the most prosperous in Haiti have not paid taxes for over forty years. In 1999, the Préval government said they were cracking down, but tax revenues have not increased notably.

8. To sweeten prospects for future investors while maintaining poor wage conditions, Washington announced during 1995 that the Overseas Private Investment Corporation (OPIC), a government agency, will provide 100 million dollars in incentives for firms wanting to do business in Haiti over the following four years (IPS 1995).

9. I heard this report on Tropique FM during February 1994. In the days following the report every attempt was made to document the source of information but, regrettably, with no success.

10. The most recent Demographic Health Survey shows that nationally, 50 percent of all Haitian households are headed by women (EMMUS III 2000).

11. This rate is extreme within the Western Hemisphere when compared to 76/100,000 in Guatemala, 110/100,000 in Jamaica, and 120/100,000 in Brazil (United Nations 1991; UNFPA 1994; WHO 2001).

12. Male opposition to family planning, though common worldwide, is not an insurmountable problem (R. Simmons, personal communication, 1996). Citing successes in Matlab, Bangladesh, where female family planning workers were initially labeled by men as prostitutes for their community-based family planning advocacy, Simmons claims, "Good programs can overcome these attitudes." I would argue that in Haiti, men's acceptance of family planning would require not only strategic family planning program interventions but also, as an obligatory prerequisite to programmatic change, a much deeper understanding of power, paternity, reproduction, and child nurturing.

CHAPTER 4. THE FAMILY PLANNING CENTER: A CLINIC IN CONFLICT

1. Trouillot (1995b:125) notes that "urbanites . . . often refer to rural dwellers as *moun andeyò* (outsiders) . . . [though] few have bothered to ask how or why rural people can be *moun andeyò* in a country that is 70 percent rural." The concept of being an "outsider" is reinforced in the clinic.

2. Todd (1989:15) notes that studies in the United States reveal that the average doctor visit lasts 15.4 minutes, more than seven times longer than the average visit in the Cité Soleil clinic. Still, Todd argues, this does not allow much time to deliver a diagnosis, prognosis, and treatment—or to elicit a patient's views on his or her problem.

3. The clinic generally provides women with one packet of pills and asks them to return each month in order to continue with the method; this is commonly referred to as "resupply."

4. The most common side effect from Norplant is change in the menstrual bleeding pattern. Irregularities range from woman to woman and may include prolonged menstrual bleeding, spotting between menstrual periods, or no bleeding at all.

CHAPTER 5. A COMMUNITY CONSUMED: FIRE, POLITICS, AND HEALTH CARE

1. I asked residents to compare the costs of food before and after the coup d'état and embargo in order to verify the increases. Some examples follow, where the first cost is before 1991, the second cost is post-1991. Most measures are in *mamit* (equivalent of a coffee can) full of rice (Hg12/Hg211), corn (Hg6/Hg19), black beans (Hg12/Hg40), red

beans (Hg15–18/Hg50), single chicken (Hg20/Hg125), sugar (Hg12 g/Hg25), and one gallon of cooking oil (Hg20 g/Hg50).

2. The nuns (primarily from Belgium) worked closely with the CDS general director and have done so for decades. One of the most poignant moments of fieldwork occurred when I was standing with a crowd, mourning the death of a political activist who had been assassinated. We all had known him well. His body was left in plain view on the main marketing road of Cité Soleil. In the midst of enormous grief shared among the observers, including the victim's wife, who was in shock, the nuns sped by in a large new jeep, their chauffeur honking the horn to disperse the crowd.

3. Indigenous healers, and therefore their clients, perceive fever as an illness rather than a symptom of an illness, according to Bernard et al. (1993).

4. I suspect that during surveys, people were too embarrassed to admit that they would rather not pay. Garnering information about anything economic is difficult in Haiti. Building rapport during qualitative interviews achieved more trust and probably more validity.

5. I employ the term "indirect costs" broadly here to explain costs that include necessary care outside of that offered in the family planning center.

6. In 1991, Vice President Dan Quayle, his wife Marilyn, and their daughter visited Haiti. As an American who knew Cité Soleil, I was asked by officials to assist the Marilyn Quayle entourage on her "urban" tour, while her husband met with Haitian officials.

7. Nag (1989) documents how investigations in Nigeria (Okediji 1975) and Kerala, India (Panikar 1979), indicate that literacy and education increase awareness not only of the need but also of the right to use health facilities.

8. The former clinic director at the Leogane site indicated that over a two-year period, fewer than 1 percent of Norplant users had the method removed. Canham-Clyne and Cooley-Prost (1996) indicate that a California study of Norplant acceptability, by contrast, revealed that nearly half of the North American women had their implants removed within two years.

9. Pèpè in the title of this booklet translates as: "coming from the United States and unnatural" in that it does not conform to the Haitian culture or context. The origin of pèpè comes from rad pèpè, second-hand or used clothing from the United States, delivered in large containers. Today, one frequently hears about demokrasi pèpè.

10. Among conservative bishops in Haiti and Rome, Aristide was not a popular priest (cf. Wilentz 1989). Steps to excommunicate him first began in 1988. He formally resigned from the priesthood after his return to Haiti in October 1994.

11. In fact, Depo-Provera does have a tainted past and is associated with dogs. Studies in the early 1970s showed that breast cancers were found in beagles treated for more than three years with Depo-Provera injections. However, the dose was equal to twenty-five times that of the human contraceptive dose, and since beagles are considerably smaller than human females the study was discounted by the FDA. The FDA claimed that beagles were not "appropriate animal models" for determining Depo-Provera side effects (Rosenthal 1999).

12. The most notable trial occurred in July 1991 against the infamous tonton makout Roger Lafontant for his January 1991 attempted coup against the legitimate democratic government. The period during the trial was declared a national holiday. Lafontant was found guilty, with hard labor for life as punishment.

CHAPTER 6.   THE POLITICAL ECONOMY OF INTERNATIONAL AID:
GROUNDING ETHNOGRAPHY, ENGAGING HISTORY

1. The role of international aid in maintaining illegitimate Haitian governments, notably the long reign of the Duvaliers, has been noted by many scholars (Trouillot 1990; Farmer 2002). Most remarkable has been the U.S. role in supporting the Duvalier's infamous graft—both Papa Doc (1957–1971) and Baby Doc (1971–1986)—through international "aid" mechanisms (Ferguson 1987; Nicholls 1979). The International Monetary Fund (IMF), for example, in 1980 gave Baby Doc's Haiti US$22 million and "within weeks US$20 million of this amount had been withdrawn from the Haitian government's account: of this, the IMF stated, US$4 million had gone to the VSN [tonton makout-s], while the remaining US$16 million had seemingly disappeared into Duvalier's various personal accounts" (Ferguson, quoted in Schuller 2003:25).

2. Years later, when I met Murray at the Applied Anthropology meetings in Albuquerque in 1993, he indicated that he hadn't stayed in "family planning" for long because it was "way too political." None of the suggestions in his paper were applied; his doctoral thesis was on agroforestry in Haiti.

3. Family-planning experiences around the world varied, depending on local and global economic influences. In Latin America, public services were initiated in Mexico in 1974, and by 1978 public services accounted for 42 to 48 percent of the births averted; Colombia also noted success by the mid-1970s with its emerging demand for fertility limitation (Potter et al. 1976). African programs, started in the late 1960s and 1970s, faced weak demand for contraception but by the late 1980s showed some success, especially in Kenya and Zimbabwe (World Bank 1993a, UNDP 2003). In Asia, payoff for the United States government and economy has been high. Early family planning investment in South Korea, Taiwan, Thailand, and Indonesia has moved these countries with formerly high fertility rates and poor economies to low fertility countries who make up a critical part of the U.S. economy and job market (PAI 2001:1).

4. In a recent study of 116 different countries, Ross et al. (2000) note that while the agenda for heavy promotion of vertical programming has been refined in the past few decades to include couples and emphasize quality, still in many parts of the world, especially where fertility has not dropped, programs continue to focus on targeted fertility levels.

5. There are some exceptions to this, of course. Pathfinder, a U.S.-based reproductive health agency with a field office in Haiti, for example, indicates that it had worked closely with the Ministry of Population and Health to reduce maternal mortality through postabortion care in public-health–sector hospitals. This type of collaboration is not common, however.

6. Haiti's government has not fully recovered from internal political strife, most notably since Prime Minister Smarth resigned in June of 1997 under President Préval. As of January 1999, the Haitian legislature had not approved a subsequent prime minister (PM), who technically and legally forms the cabinet. Hence any laws or policies proposed by the government cannot be passed or accepted as truly "official." The Aristide administration, prior to the coup of February 2004, voted to appoint a PM, but the current PM has not been approved for lack of quorum. This issue was a long-standing and deeply political debate in Haiti that questioned the validity of the May 2000 elections.

7. Germain (2003:3): "The Global Gag Rule is devastating the operations of family planning clinics and women's health services around the world, and has left some

communities with no health care provision at all—at a time when more than 500,000 women die from pregnancy-related causes and over a million women die from AIDS annually. The Gag Rule has hit Africa especially hard. Lesotho, where 25 percent of women are infected with HIV/AIDS, no longer receives U.S.AID contraceptives following the refusal of the country's major family planning organization to agree to the Gag Rule restrictions. In Ghana, nearly 700,000 clients no longer have access to HIV prevention services, which were cut because NGO healthcare providers there lost U.S.AID funding under Gag Rule strictures."

8. The 1994 Cairo agreement shifted the world's approach to reducing rapid population growth away from coercive programs with quotas to voluntary family-planning programs that at their core were about empowering women to make choices and have control over their lives.

9. Congressional supporters of UNFPA objected and blocked USAID from spending the funds Congress had earmarked for UNFPA, hoping that UNFPA might again be judged eligible to receive a U.S. contribution in the future. Although there was some initial confusion about whether family planning was to be included, of the total of US$34 million proposed to be reprogrammed to Afghanistan and Pakistan, two-thirds is for family planning, one-third for other maternal health activities (personal communication, Craig Lascher 2003).

CHAPTER 7. HEALTH IN HAITI: PRODUCING EQUITY

1. Ross and Frankenberg (1993:2) indicate that "changes in contraceptive prevalence and fertility can be related: a 15 point increase in contraceptive prevalence implies that the total fertility rate may fall about one child." The nearly doubling of the contraceptive rate in Haiti, however, has had no substantial impact on the total fertility rate.

2. Singer and Castro's (2004:xvi) recent definition of CMA demonstrates how the political economy framework, as I have applied it, is virtually identical to the CMA perspective. The CMA perspective (1) recognizes that health itself is a profoundly political issue, one that often is contentious if not explosive; (2) is cognizant and critical of the colonial heritage of anthropology and the tendency of conventional medical anthropology to serve as a "handmaiden of biomedicine"; (3) balances concern for unbiased social science with an awareness of the sociohistoric origin and political nature of all scientific knowledge; (4) acknowledges the fundamental importance of class, racial, and sexual inequity in determining the distribution of health, disease, living and working conditions, and health care; (5) defines power as a fundamental variable in health-related research, policy, and programming; (6) avoids the artificial separation of local settings and micropopulations from their wider political-economic contexts; (7) asserts that its mission is emancipatory: it aims not simply to understand but also to change culturally inappropriate, oppressive, and exploitative patterns in the health arena and beyond; and (8) sees commitment to change as fundamental to the discipline.

3. The zone is not quite as isolated as Cité Soleil.

4. Fonkoze currently has 25,000 loan clients, 96 percent of whom are women (Fonkoze 2004).

5. When it was first initiated, PPFA legally challenged the Mexico City policy, also known as the Global Gag Rule, discussed in chapter 6. When the court rejected PPFA's constitutional claims in September 1990, USAID terminated PPFA-I's eligibility for population funds. Two affiliates to the international branch of PPFA, including the

Miami-based Caribbean and Latin America office, raised private funds to make up funding lost through USAID. Although PPFA-I is regularly cited as promoting abortion services in the countries where it funds programs (Scott 2005), both APROSIFA and ZL have never provided any abortion-related services.

6. I did not interview any *manbo-s*, or Voudou priestesses, but they too could provide these services.

BIBLIOGRAPHY

Abernathy, V. n.d. The Demographic Transition Revisited: Lessons for Foreign Aid and U.S. Immigration Policy. Nashville, Tenn.: Vanderbilt University School of Medicine, Department of Psychiatry. http://www.carryingcapacity.org/va2.html.

Adams, V. 1998. *Doctors for Democracy: Health Professionals in the Nepal Revolution*. New York: Cambridge University Press.

Adrien, A., and M. Cayemittes. 1991. Le Sida en Haïti: Connaissances, attitudes, croyances, et comportements de la population. Port-au-Prince: Bureau de Coordination du Programme National de Lutte Contre le Sida, January.

Ali, K. 2002. *Planning the Family in Egypt: New Bodies, New Selves*. Austin: University of Texas Press.

Allman, J. 1980. Sexual Unions in Rural Haiti. *International Journal of Sociology and the Family* 10:15–39.

Altman, D. 2001. *Global Sex*. Chicago: University of Chicago Press.

Alvarez, M., and G. Murray. 1981. Socialization for Scarcity: Child Feeding Beliefs and Practices in a Haitian Village. Unpublished Report, submitted to USAID/HAITI, Port-au-Prince, 28 August.

America's Watch Committee (US) and National Coalition for Haitian Refugees. 1993. *Silencing a People: The Destruction of Civil Society in Haiti*. New York: Human Rights Watch.

Anagnost, A. 1995. A Surfeit of Bodies: Population and the Rationality of the State in Post-Mao-China. In *Conceiving the New World Order: The Global Politics of Reproduction*, edited by F. Ginsburg and R. Rapp, Berkeley: University of California Press.

APROSIFA (Association for the Promotion of Integrated Family Health). 2003. *Rapport annuel*. Port-au-Prince.

Aristide, J. B. 1994. Women in Labor for Deliverance. Message of the President. Unpublished manuscript. Washington, D.C.: Government of Haiti, 23 July, i–ii.

Associated Press. 1993a. Haiti Slum Burned after Mob Kills 2 Officials. *The Grand Rapids Press*, 30 December, 4.

———. 1993b. U.S. Providing $100,000 to Aid 5,000 Left Homeless in Port-au-Prince Slum Fire. *The Grand Rapids Press*, 30 December, 4.

Auguste, R. 1995. Health, Population, and Family Planning. *Roots* 1(3):13–20.

Augustin, A., and M. Gay. 1991. Rapport d'enquête: Abandon des méthodes contraceptives. Port-au-Prince: IPPF/PAPFO and IHE, January.

Baer, H., M. Singer, and I. Susser, eds. 1997. *Medical Anthropology and the World System: A Critical Perspective*. Westport, Conn.: Bergin and Garvey.

Ballweg, J. A., R. E. Webb, and G. Biamby. 1974. Mortality and the Acceptability of Family Planning in a Haitian Community. *Community Health* 5(6):306–311.

Banque Mondiale. 1979. Haïti: Etude du secteur urbain. Rapport no. 2152. Bureau Régional de l'Amérique Latine et des Antilles: Département des Programmes I, Port-au-Prince.

Batliwala, S. 1994. The Meaning of Women's Empowerment: New Concepts from Action. In *Population Policies Reconsidered: Health, Empowerment and Rights*, edited by G. Sen, A. Germain, and L. C. Chen. Boston: Harvard School of Public Health.

Becker, A. 1985. Choice of Location for Childbirth in Cité Simone, Haiti. Unpublished manuscript, Complexe Medico-Social de la Cité Simone and the Department of Social Medicine and Health Policy, Harvard Medical School, Cambridge.

Behets, F. 2003. Policy Profile: Haitians Reach Consensus on National STD Guidelines. AIDS Captions. Family Health International. http://www.fhi.org/en/HIVAIDS/Publications/Archive/articles/AIDScaptions/volume3no1/HaitianConsensus.htm.

Behets, F. M., J. Desormeaux, D. Joseph, M. Adrien, G. Coicou, G. Dallabetta, H. A. Hamilton, S. Moeng, H. Davis, M. S. Cohen, and R. Boulos. 1995. Control of Sexually Transmitted Diseases in Haiti: Results and Implications of a Baseline Study among Pregnant Women Living in Cité Soleil Shantytowns. *Journal of Infectious Diseases* 172:764–771.

Bell, B. 1995. Women's Struggles, Women's Hopes. Unpublished manuscript, Washington, D.C.: International Liaison Office for President Aristide.

———. 2001. *Walking on Fire: Haitian Women's Stories of Survival and Resistance*. Ithaca: Cornell University Press.

Bernard, J. B., G. de Zalduondo, M. L. Mayard, N. Phelle, E. St. Louis, M. Saint Louis, and R. Abellard. 1993. *L'Insalubrité dans les bidonvilles: Le cas de Cité-Soleil*. Paper presented at the Association of American Anthropologists, Washington D.C., November.

Black, I. 2002. EU Replaces Cash Denied to UN Family Planning by US. *The Guardian*, 24 July.

Blanc, A. 2001. The Effect of Power in Sexual Relationships on Sexual and Reproductive Health: An Examination of the Evidence. *Studies in Family Planning* 32(3):189.

Bledsoe, C., A. G. Hill, U. D'Allessandro, and P. Langerock. 1994. Constructing Natural Fertility: The Use of Western Contraceptive Technologies in Rural Gambia. *Population and Development Review* 20(1):81–113.

Bohning, D. 1996. Many of Haiti's Poorest Will Soon Lose a Lifeline. *Miami Herald*, 14 April, 1, 21.

Bongaarts, J., and J. Bruce. 1995. The Causes of Unmet Need for Contraception and the Social Content of Services. *Studies in Family Planning* 26(2):57–75.

Bongaarts, J., and S. C. Watkins. 1996. Social Interactions and Contemporary Fertility Transitions. *Population and Development Review* 22(4):639–682.

Bordes, A. 1981a. We Must Take Time . . . *People* 8(2):5.

———. 1981b. *L'Importance des resultats de l'enquête haïtienne sur la fécondité pour l'elaboration d'une planification familiale pour Haïti*. Port-au-Prince: Institut Haïtien de Statistique et d'Informatique.

Bordes, A., and A. Couture. 1978. *For the People, For a Change*. Boston: Beacon.

Boulos, M., R. Boulos, and D. Nichols. 1991. Perceptions and Practices Relating to Condom Use among Urban Men in Haiti. *Studies in Family Planning* 22(5):318–325.

Boulos, R. 1985. Operations Research to Improve Access and Continuation of Family Planning through Community Based Outreach in Cité Simone, an Urban Slum of Port-au-Prince, Haiti. Final Report. New York: Center for Population and Family Health, Columbia University.

Boulos, R., J. Pierre-Louis, and J. Tafforeau. 1986. Contraceptive Continuation Rates. The Family Planning Center, Medical Social Complex of Cité Simone. Unpublished report.

Boulos, R., N. Halsey, E. Holt, A. Ruff, J. R. Brutus, T. C. Quinn, M. Adrien, C. Boulos. 1990. HIV-1 in Haitian Women 1982–1988. The Cité Soleil /JHU AIDS Project Team. *Journal of Acquired Immune Deficiency Syndrome* 3(7):721–728.

Boulos, R., A. Ruff, A. Hahmias, E. Holt, et al. 1992. Herpes Simplex Virus Type 2 Infection, Syphilis, and Hepatitis B Virus Infection in Haitian Women with Human Immunodeficiency Virus Type 1 and Human T Lymphotropic Virus Type I Infections. *Journal of Infectious Diseases* 166(2):418–420.

Brodwin, P. 1996. *Medicine and Morality in Haiti: The Concept for Healing Power.* New York: Cambridge University Press.

Browner, C. H., and C. F. Sargent. 1996. Anthropology and Studies of Human Reproduction. In *Handbook of Medical Anthropology Contemporary Theory and Method*, revised edition, edited by C. F. Sargent and T. M. Johnson. Westport, Conn.: Greenwood Press.

Bruce, J. 1989. Fundamental Elements of the Quality of Care: A Simple Framework. Working Papers no. 1. New York: Population Council.

Bruce, J., C. B. Lloyd, and A. Leonard, with P. Engle and N. Duffy. 1995. *Families in Focus: New Perspectives on Mothers, Fathers, and Children.* New York: Population Council.

Brutus, J. 1989. *Seroprévalence de HIV parmi les femmes enceintes à Cité Soleil, Haïti.* Paper presented at the Fifth International Conference on AIDS, Montreal.

Brydon, L., and S. Chant. 1993. *Women in the Third World.* Reprint, Aldershot: Edward Elgar.

Burns, A., R. Lovich, J. Maxwell, K. Shapiro, and J. Steve. 2000. *Kote Fanm Pa Jwenn Doktè: Yon Gid Santé pou Fanm.* Berkeley: Hesperian Foundation.

Burton, N. 1989. Midterm Evaluation Private Sector Family Planning Project (PSFP). Report prepared for the Human Resources Office, Population Section. Port-au-Prince: USAIF/Haiti and IPPF Western Hemisphere Region.

———. 1993. Recommendations for Consolidation of Activities. Memorandum. Port-au-Prince: CDS Family Planning Program, USAID.

Caceres, C. 2000. The Production of Knowledge on Sexuality in the Era of AIDS. In *Framing the Sexual Subject: The Politics of Gender, Sexuality and Power*, edited by R. G. Parker, R. M. Barbosa, and P. Aggleton. Berkeley: University of California Press.

Cain, M. T. 1981. Risk and Insurance: Perspectives on Fertility and Agrarian Change in India and Bangladesh. *Population and Development Review* 7(3):435–474.

Caldwell, J. 1997. The Global Fertility Transition: The Need for a Unifying Theory. *Population and Development Review* 23(4):803–812.

Campbell, C. 2003. *Letting Them Die: Why HIV/AIDS Intervention Programmes Fail.* Wetton, South Africa: Double Story Books.

Canham-Clyne, J., and W. Cooley-Prost. 1996. "U.S. AID Go Home!" In *Third World Traveler.* http://www.thirdworldtraveler.com/US_ThirdWorld/AID_Haiti.html.

CARE-International. 1990. Multi-Year Plan: July 1990–June 1995. Unpublished document. Port-au-Prince.

CARE-International Haiti. 1993. FY 1993 Project Implementation and Evaluation (PIE) Report for RICHES. Submitted by S. Igras for the period July–December 1992. Port-au-Prince.

Caritas of Haiti. 1986. Message of Caritas National for International Women's Day. Women's Promotion Branch. Papye-Hinche, 8 March.

Carter, A. 2001. Social Processes and Fertility Change: Anthropological Perspectives. In *Diffusion Processes and Fertility Transition: Selected Perspectives.* Washington, D.C.: National Academy Press.

Castro, A. 2004. Contracepting at Childbirth: The Integration of Reproductive Health and Population Policies in Mexico. In *Unhealthy Health Policy: A Critical Anthropological Examination*, edited by A. Castro and M. Singer, 133–144. Walnut Creek, Cal.: Altamira Press.

Castro A., A. Heimburger, and A. Langer. 2002. *Iatrogenic Epidemic: How Health Care Professionals Contribute to the High Proportion of Cesarean Sections in Mexico.* Working Papers on Latin America, no. 02/03–3. Cambridge: David Rockefeller Center for Latin American Studies at Harvard University.

Cayemittes, M., and A. Chahnazarian. 1989. *Survie et santé de l'enfant en Haïti: Résultats de l'enquête moralité, morbidité et utilisation des services 1987.* Port-au-Prince: Institut Haïtien de l'Enfance, Ministère de la Santé Publique et de la Population et Johns Hopkins University.

CDS (Centres pour le Developpement et la Santé). 1993. Preliminary Results: STD Study. Unpublished study results.

——. 1996. *Point de Presse.* 31 Mars.

Center for Health and Gender Equity. 2004. International Family Planning and the Global Gag Rule. In *The 4th Global Scorecard on the Bush Administration.* http://www.globalscorecard.org.

Chahnazarian, A. 1991. *Hausse récente de la fecondité en Haiti: Un nouvel engouement pour la vie en union.* Johns Hopkins Population Center Working Paper no. 91–03. Baltimore: Johns Hopkins University.

Chanel, I. M. 1993. Population: For Many Haitian Women, Childbirth Means Death. *InterPress Service,* no date. http://www.aegis.org/news/ips/1997/IP971202.html.

——. 1997. HEALTH–AIDS: Condom Use in Haiti Relates to Income Levels. *InterPress Service,* 4 December. http://www.aegis.org/news/ips/1997/IP971202.html.

CHI/CDC (Child Health Institute and the Centers for Disease Control Division of Reproductive Health). 1991. *Haiti National Contraceptive Prevalence Survey 1989.* Atlanta: U.S. Department of Health and Human Services.

CIA (Central Intelligence Agency). 2005. Haiti: Rank Order, Total Fertility Rate. CIA Factbook, 2005. http://www.cia.gov/cia/publications/factbook/rankorder/2127rank.html.

CIAFD (Comité Inter-Agences Femmes et Developpement). 1991. *La situation des femmes haïtiennes.* Port-au-Prince: CIAFD-Système des Nations Unies.

Colon, S. 1976. The Traditional Use of Medicinal Plants and Herebs in the Province of Pedernales, Santo Domingo. *Ethnomedicine* 4:139–166.

Comaroff, J. 1985. *Body of Power, Spirit of Resistance.* Chicago: University of Chicago Press.

Concannon, B., Jr. 2002. Emmanuel Constant 2002. Haiti Solidarity Week Packet. *The Haiti Reborn.* A Program of the Quixote Center. 3–10 January.

Cook, R. 1972. *The Year of the Intern.* New York: New American Library.

Cordell, D., and J. W. Gregory., eds. 1987. *African Population and Capitalism: Historical Perspectives.* Madison: University of Wisconsin Press.

Coreil, J., P. Losikoff, R. Pincu, G. Mayard, A. J. Ruff, J. P. Hausler, J. Desmoreau, H. Davis, R. Boulos, and N. Halsey. 1998. Cultural Feasibility Studies in Preparation for Clinical Trials to Reduce Maternal-Infant HIV Transmission in Haiti. *AIDS Education and Prevention* 10(1):46–62.

Correa, S. 1994. *Population and Reproductive Rights: Feminist Perspectives from the South.* London: Zed Books.

——. 2000. Commentaries in *Culture, Health, and Sexuality* 2(3):339–343.

Correa, S., and R. Petchesky. 1994. Reproductive and Sexual Rights: A Feminist Perspective. In *Population Policies Reconsidered: Health, Empowerment and Rights,* edited by G. Sen, A. Germain and L. C. Chen. Boston: Harvard School of Public Health.

Country Reports on Human Rights Practices. 2002. Released by the Bureau of Democracy, Human Rights, and Labor, 31 March, 2003. Washington, D.C.

Curtin, P. 1990. *The Rise and Fall of the Plantation Complex.* Cambridge: Cambridge University Press.

Davis-Floyd, R. 2004. Home Birth Emergencies in the United States: The Trouble with Transport. In *Unhealthy Health Policy: A Critical Anthropological Examination,* edited by A. Castro and M. Singer, Walnut Creek, Cal.: Altamira Press.

De Brun, S. and R. H. Elling. 1987. Cuba and the Philippines: Contrasting Cases in World-System Analysis. *International Journal of Health Services* 17(4):681–701.

de Zalduondo, B. O. 1991. Culture, Health and Sexuality: Reducing HIV Risk in Haiti. Department of Health and Human Services, Public Health Service. Unpublished manuscript. Johns Hopkins University.

de Zalduondo, B. O., J. Bernard, and the Culture, Health and Sexuality Project Team. 1995. Meanings and Consequences of Sexual Economic Exchange: Gender, Poverty, and Sexual Risk Behavior in Urban Haiti. In *Conceiving Sexuality: Approaches to Sex Research in a Post-Modern World*, edited by R. Parker and J. Gagnon. New York: Rutledge Press.

Demeny, P. 1988. Social Science and Population Policy. *Population and Development Review* 14(3):451–479.

de St. Mery, M. 1958. *Description topographique, physique, civile, politique, et histoire de la patrie française de l'Isle Saint-Domingue (1797–1798)*. 3 vols. (new ed., B. Maurel and E. Taillemite, eds.). Paris: Société de l'Histoire des Colonies Françaises and Librairie Larousse.

Despagne, P. 1988. Projet de recherche operationnelle, Centres pour le Développement et la Santé. In Planification familiale rapport d'activités du Centre de PF. Port-au-Prince: CDS.

Desvarieux, M., P. R. Hyppolite, and J. W. Pape. 2001. A Novel Approach to Directly Observed Therapy for Tuberculosis in an HIV-Endemic Area. *American Journal of Public Health* 91(1):138–141.

DHS–I Surveys. 1985/90. *Demographic and Health Surveys*. Columbia, Md.: Institute for Resource Development/Macro Systems, Inc.

Di Leonardo, M. 1991. Gender, Culture, and Political Economy: Feminist Anthropology in Historical Perspective. In *Gender at the Crossroads of Knowledge: Feminist Anthropology in the Postmodern Era*, edited by M. di Leonardo. Berkeley: University of California Press.

Dixon-Mueller, R. 1993. The Sexuality Connection in Reproductive Health. *Studies in Family Planning* 24(5):269–282.

Dixon-Mueller, R., and A. Germain. 2000. Reproductive Health and the Demographic Imagination. In *Women's Empowerment and Demographic Processes: Moving beyond Cairo*, edited by H. Presser and G. Sen. Oxford: Oxford University Press.

Dowell, S., H. Davis, et al. 1993. The Utility of Verbal Autopsies for Identifying HIV–1 Related Deaths in Haitian Children. *AIDS* 7:1255–1259.

Doyal, L. 1995. *What Makes Women Sick: Gender and the Political Economy of Health*. New Brunswick: Rutgers University Press.

———. 2000. Gender Equity in Health: Debates and Dilemmas. *Social Science and Medicine* 51(6):931–939.

The Economist. 2002. Economic Focus: Does Population Matter? *Economist*, 7 December, 74.

Ellen, R. 2002. "Déjà Vu, All Over Again", Again: Reinvention and Progress in Applying Local Knowledge to Development. In *Participating in Development: Approaches to Indigenous Knowledge*, Edited by P. Sillitoe, A. Bicker, and J. Pottier. London: Routledge.

EMMUS I. 1987. *Enquête mortalité, morbidité et utilisation des services, Haiti*. Calverton, Md.: Ministère de la Santé Publique et de la Population, Institut Haitien de l'Enfance et ORC Macro.

EMMUS II. 1994–1995. *Enquête mortalité, morbidité et utilisation des services, Haiti*. Calverton, Md.: Ministère de la Santé Publique et de la Population, Institut Haitien de l'Enfance et ORC Macro.

EMMUS III. 2000. *Enquête mortalité, morbidité et utilisation des services, Haiti.* Calverton, Md.: Ministère de la Santé Publique et de la Population, Institut Haitien de l'Enfance et ORC Macro.

FAO (Food and Agriculture Organization). 2001. Part III. Latin America and the Caribbean. In *The State of Food and Agriculture.* Regional Overview. http://www.fao.org/docrep/003/x9800e/x9800e10.htm.

Farah, D. 1994. Haiti's Tiny Victims. *Washington Post,* 30 June, A1.

Farmer, P. 1988a. Bad Blood, Spoiled Milk: Bodily Fluids as Moral Barometers in Rural Haiti. *American Ethnologist* 15:62–83.

———. 1988b. Blood, Sweat, and Baseballs: Haiti in the West Atlantic System. *Dialectical Anthropology* 13:83–99.

———. 1990a. Sending Sickness: Sorcery, Politics, and Changing Concepts of AIDS in Rural Haiti. *Medical Anthropology Quarterly* 4(1):6–27.

———. 1990b. AIDS and Accusation: Haiti, Haitians, and the Geography of Blame. In *Cultural Aspects of AIDS: The Human Factor,* edited by D. Feldman. New York: Praeger.

———. 1994. *The Uses of Haiti.* Monroe, Maine: Common Courage Press.

———. 1995. The Significance of Haiti. In *Haiti, Dangerous Crossroads. North American Congress on Latin America (NACLA),* edited by D. McFaden, P. LaRamée, M. Fried, and F. Rosen. Boston: South End Press.

———. 1999. *Infections and Inequalities: The Modern Plagues.* Berkeley: University of California Press.

———. 2002. Introducing ARVs in Resource-Poor Settings: Expected and Unexpected Challenges and Consequences. Paper presented at the XIV International AIDS Conference, Barcelona, 11 July.

———. 2003. *Pathologies of Power.* Berkeley: University of California Press.

———. 2004a. Political Violence and Public Health in Haiti. *New England Journal of Medicine* 350(15):1483–1486.

———. 2004b. Haiti: Unjust Aid Embargo during Health Emergency. *Haiti Reborn News.* http://www.haitireborn.org/campaigns/lhl/unjust-aid-embarg-p-farmer.php#_ednref10.

Farmer, P., M. Connors, and J. Simmons, eds. 1997. *Women, Poverty and AIDS: Sex, Drugs, and Structural Violence.* Boston: Common Courage Press.

Farmer, P., and M. C. Smith Fawzi. 2002. Unjust Embargo Deepens Haiti's Health Crisis. Op-ed, *Boston Globe,* 30 December. http://www/pih.org/inthenews/021230farmersmithoped.htm.

Fass, S. 1980. The Economics of Survival: A Study of Poverty and Planning in Haiti. Office of Urban Development, Bureau for Development Support. Unpublished manuscript, Washington, D.C.: Agency for International Development – International Development Cooperation Agency.

———. 1988. *Political Economy in Haiti: The Drama of Survival.* New Brunswick, N.J.: Transaction.

Fatahalla, M. F. 1994. Fertility Control Technology: A Women-Centered Approach to Research. In *Population Policies Reconsidered: Health, Empowerment and Rights,* Edited by G. Sen, A. Germain, and L. C. Chen. Boston: Harvard School of Public Health.

Fatton, R., Jr. 2002. *Haiti's Predatory Republic: The Unending Transition to Democracy.* Boulder, Col.: Lynne Rienner.

Feminist Daily New Wire. 2002a. Bush Makes UNFPA Funding Cut Official. 23 July. http://www.feminist.org/news/newsbyte/uswirestory.asp?id=6723.

———. 2002b. US to Back away from UN Population Policy. 4 Nov. http://www.feminist.org/news/newsbyte/uswirestory.asp?id=7248.

Ferguson, J. 1987. *Papa Doc, Baby Doc: Haiti and the Duvaliers.* Oxford: Basil Blackwell.

———. 1994. *The Anti-Politics Machine: Development, Depoliticization, and Bureaucratic Power in Lesotho.* Minneapolis: University of Minnesota Press.

Ferguson, J. 1999. Country Profile: Haiti. *New Internationalist,* issue 316, http://www. newintorg/issue316/profile.htm

Fick, C. 1990. *The Making of Haiti: The Saint Domingue Revolution from Below.* Knoxville: University of Tennessee Press.

Fine, M. 1992. Passions, Politics, and Power: Feminist Research Possibilities. In *Disruptive Voices: The Possibilities of Feminist Research,* edited by M. Fine. Ann Arbor: University of Michigan Press.

Finkle, J. L., and C. A. McIntosh. 2002. United Nations Population Conferences: Shaping the Policy Agenda for the Twenty-First Century. *Studies in Family Planning* 33(1):11–23.

Firth, R. 1964. *Essays on Social Organization and Values.* London School of Economics, Monographs on Social Anthropology no. 38. New York: Athlone Press, Humanities Press.

Fisher, S., and A. D. Todd. 1986. *Discourse and Institutional Authority: Medicine, Education, and Law.* Norwood, N.J.: Ablex Publishing.

Folbre, N. 1983. Of Patriarchy Born: The Political Economy of Fertility Decisions. *Feminist Studies* 9:261–284.

Fonkoze. 2004. Three Courageous Haitian Women Save Micro-finance Bank Branch Office from Looting by Armed Rebels—Press Release. http://www.fonkoze.org/newsroom/ pressrelease3.31.04.htm.

Food First. n.d. Myth: Too Many Mouths to Feed—Good and Bad Fertility Declines http:// www.globalissues.org/EnvIssues/Population/Hunger/FoodFirst/Fertility.asp.

Foreign Policy and the Fund for Peace 2005. The Failed States Index July/August 2005. http://www.foreignpolicy.com/story/cms.php?story_id=3098.

Foucault, M. 1980. *Power/Knowledge: Selected Interviews and Other Writings, 1972–1977.* Edited by C. Gordon. Brighton, United Kingdom: Harvester.

François, A. 1995. Women's Rights and the Judicial System. *Roots* 1(3):21–25.

Fund for Peace. 2005. Failed States Index. http://www.fundforpeace.org/programs/fsi/ fsindex.php.

Gay, J. 1980. A Literature Review of the Client-Provider Interface in Maternal and Child Health and Family Planning Clinics in Latin America. Washington, D.C.: Pan-American Health Organization/World Health Organization.

Gayle, H. 2003. Introductory Notes of International Women's Day Briefing: AIDS Has a Woman's Face. Third Annual Women's Global Health Imperative. San Francisco: University of California, 7 March.

Gebrian, B. 1993. Community Participation in Primary Health Care in Rural Haiti: An Ecological Approach. PhD. dissertation, University of Connecticut.

Geitner, P. 2002. European Union to Step in with More Money for UN Population Fund after United States Withholds Funds. Center for Disease Control and Prevention International News. In *The Body: An AIDS and HIV Information Source,* Excerpted from Associated Press, 24 July. http://www.thebody.com/cdc/news_updates_archive/july24_02/ eu_population_fund.html.

George, A. 2003. Using Accountability to Improve Reproductive Health Care. *Reproductive Health Matters* 11(21):161–170.

Germain, A. 2003. A U.S.-German Dialogue on Governance and Global Health. Remarks by Adrienne Germain, 20–21 November. Unpublished document.

Ginsburg, F., and R. Rapp. 1991. The Politics of Reproduction. *Annual Review of Anthropology* 20:311–343.

———. 1995. *Conceiving the New World Order: The Global Politics of Reproduction.* Berkeley: University of California Press.

Godard, H. 1985. Port-au-Prince – Quartiers. In *Atlas Planche 11.* Bordeaux: Centre d'Etude de Géographie Tropicale and Université de Bordeaux.

Goff, S. 2000. *Hideous Dream: A Soldier's Memoir of the US Invasion in Haiti.* New York: Soft Skull Press.

Goode, E. 2003. Certain Words Can Trip up AIDS Grants. *New York Times,* 18 April, A10.

GRAIP (Groupe de Récherche et d'Appui au Initiatives Populaires). 1994. *Prospectus.* Port-au-Prince: GRAIP.

Grann, D. 2001. Giving "The Devil" His Due. *Atlantic Monthly* 287(6). http://www.theatlantic.com/issues/2001/06/grann.htm.

Green, M. 1993. The Evolution of US International Population Policy, 1965–92: A Chronological Account. *Population and Development Review* 19(2):303–321.

Greene, L. 1994. Violence to Women in Haiti Needs To Be Addressed. *Boston Herald,* October 28.

Greenhalgh, S. 1988. Fertility as Mobility: Sinic Transitions. *Population and Development Review* 14(4):629–674.

———. 1990. Toward a Political Economy of Fertility: Anthropological Contributions. *Population and Development Review* 16(1):96–106.

———. 1994. Anthropological Contributions to Fertility Theory. Working Papers no. 64. New York: Population Council.

———. 1995. *Situating Fertility.* Cambridge: Cambridge University Press.

Greenhalgh, S., and J. Li. 1995. Engendering Reproductive Policy and Practice in Peasant China: For a Feminist Demography of Reproduction. *Signs: Journal of Women in Culture and Society* 20(3):601–641.

Guengant, J., and J. May. n.d. Haiti Population Strategy Paper (1989–1990). Washington, D.C.: The Futures Group.

Gupta, G. R. 2002. How Men's Power over Women Fuels the HIV Epidemic: It Limits Women's Ability to Control Sexual Interactions. *British Medical Journal* 324(7331):183.

Gutmann, M. 1996. *The Meaning of Macho: Being a Man in Mexico City.* Berkeley: University of California Press.

Guyer, J. 1988. Dynamic Approaches to Domestic Budgeting: Cases and Methods from Africa. In *A Home Divided: Women and Income in the Third World,* edited by D. Dwyer and J. Bruce. Stanford: Stanford University Press.

Haiti Info. 1999. Fire Victims Paid Off. *Haiti Info* 6(24):3.

Haïti Progrès. 2002. Cité Soleil, <<Ville sans loi>>. *Haïti Progrès* 19(46) 30 January. http://www.haiti-progres.com/2002/sm020130/

Halsey, N. 1993. Increased Mortality after High Titer Measles Vaccines: Too Much of a Good Thing. *Pediatric Infectious Disease Journal* 12:462–465.

Halsey, N., J. Coberly, E. Holt, J. Coreil, P. Kissinger, L. Moulton, J. R. Brutus, and R. Boulos. 1992. Sexual Behavior, Smoking, and HIV–1 Infection in Haitian Women. *Journal of the American Medical Association* 267(15):2062–2066.

Halstead, B., J. Walsh, and K. Warren, eds. 1985. *Good Health at Low Cost.* New York: Rockefeller Foundation.

Hamilton-Phelan, A. 1994. The Latest Political Weapon in Haiti: Military Rapes of Women and Girls. *Los Angeles Times,* 5 June, M4.

Hammel, E. A. 1990. A Theory of Culture for Demography. *Population Development Review* 16(3):455–485.

Hammel, E. A., and D. Friou. 1997. Anthropology and Demography: Marriage, Liaison, or Encounter? In *Anthropological Demography,* edited by D. I. Kertzer and T. Fricke. Chicago: University of Chicago Press.

Handwerker, W. P. 1989. *Women's Power and Social Revolution: Fertility Transition in the West Indies.* London: Sage.

————. 1993. Gender Power Differences between Parents and High-Risk Sexual Behavior by Their Children: AIDS/STD Risk Factors Extend to a Prior Generation. *Journal of Women's Health* 2(3):301–316.

Hardon, A., and E. Hayes. 1997. *Reproductive Rights in Practice: A Feminist Report of Quality of Care.* Houndmills, Hampshire, U.K.: London: Zed.

Hartmann, B. 1995. *Reproductive Rights and Wrongs: The Global Politics of Population Control.* Rev. ed. Boston: South End Press.

————. 1997. Population Control I: Birth of an Ideology. *International Journal of Health Services* 27:523–540.

Heise, L., K. Moore, and N. Toubia. 1995. *Sexual Coercion and Reproductive Health: A Focus on Research.* New York: Population Council.

Heise, L., J. Pitangy, and A. Germain. 1994. Violence against Women: The Hidden Health Burden. World Bank Discussion Papers no. 255. Washington, D.C.: World Bank.

Helzner, J. F. 2002. Transforming Family Planning Services in the Latin American and Caribbean Region. *Studies in Family Planning* 33(1):49–60.

Hirsch, J. 2003. *A Courtship after Marriage: Sexuality and Love in Mexican Transnational Families.* Berkeley: University of California Press.

Holt, E., L. Moulron, et al. 1993. Differential Mortality by Measles Vaccine Titer and Sex. *Journal of Infectious Diseases* 168:1087–1096.

Human Rights Watch. 2002. *World Report 2002/Haiti.* http://www.hrw.org/wr2k2/americas.html.

Human Rights Watch/National Coalition for Haitian Refugees. 1994. Terror Prevails in Haiti: Human Rights Violations and Failed Diplomacy. Washington, D.C. and New York vol. 6, no. 5, April. http://hrw.org/doc/?t=americas.backgrounder&c=haiti.

IDB (Inter American Development Bank). 1990. Economic and Social Progress in Latin America: 1990 Report. (Special section: Working Women in Latin America.) Washington, D.C.

IHS/WFS (Institut Haïtien de statistique et Enquête Mondial sur La Fecondité). 1981. *Enquête haïtienne sur la fecondité (1977).* Rapport national vol 1. London.

Inhorn, M., and Van Balen, F., eds. 2002. *Infertility around the Globe: New Thinking on Childlessness, Gender and Reproductive Technologies.* Berkeley and Los Angeles: University of California Press.

INHSAC (Institut Haitien de Santé Communautaire). http://www.inhsac.org.

Inter-American Commission on Human Rights. 1988. Report on the Situation of Human Rights in Haiti, chapter 2, Political Rights. Organization of American States (OAS)/ Ser.L/V/II.74, doc. 9 rev. 17 September. http://www.cidh.oas.org/countryrep/ Haiti88eng/chap.2c.htm.

Inter-American Development Bank, European Commission, the United Nations and the World Bank. 2004. Summary Report, Haiti: Interim Cooperation Framework 2004–2006, Cadre de Cooperation Interimaire Haiti, July.

IPPF (International Planned Parenthood Federation). 2001. "Haiti: Development of Management and Logistics Resources to Improve Quality of Care" Notes from the Field no. 2 (Published 2001.04). http://ippfwhr.org/publications/serial_issue_e.asp?PubID= 34&SerialIssuesID=75.

IPS (InterPress Service). 1995. Haiti-US: Clinton Announces Visit to Haiti as IMF Grants Loan. *InterPress Service.* Distribution via APC networks, 9 March.

Ives, K. 1995. The Lavalas Alliance Propels Aristide to Power. In *Haiti, Dangerous Crossroads,* edited by D. McFadyen, L. Pierre, M. Fried and F. Rosen. North American Congress on Latin America (NACLA). Boston, Mass.: South End Press.

Jacob, J. 1987. Protocole d'étude socio-anthropologique sur la faible utilisation des sterilets par les femmes de la Cité Soleil, Port-au-Prince. Port-au-Prince: CSCMS. Cité Soleil Centre Medico-Sociale.

James, C.L.R. 1989. *The Black Jacobians*. 3rd. ed. New York: Vintage Books.

JHPIEGO. 2000. Quality of Care Conference in Haiti. JHPIEGO. TrainerNews. http://www.reproline.jhu.edu.

Kabeer, N. 1994. *Reversed Realities: Gender Hierarchies in Development Thought*. New York: Verso.

Kaler, A. 2004a. The Moral Lens of Population Control: Condoms and Controversies in Southern Malawi. *Studies in Family Planning* 35(2):n.p.

———. 2004b. The Female Condom in North America: Selling the Technology of Empowerment. *Journal of Gender Studies* 13(2):n.p.

Kamber, M. 2004. Haiti's Political Vacuum Stokes Flames of Gang Violence. Port-au-Prince Journal. *New York Times*, International Section, 2 November.

Kane, T., F. Gaston, and B. Janowitz. 1990. Initial Acceptability of Contraceptive Implants in Four Developing Countries. *International Family Planning Perspectives* 16(2):49–54.

Kennedy, M., and D. Williams. 1995. Ending Violence against Women in Haiti: Toward a Democratic Recovery. Report of HAITIwoman Conference, Cambridge, Mass.: I, II.

Kertzer, D. I., and T. Fricke. 1997. Toward an Anthropological Demography. In *Anthropological Demography*, edited by D. I. Kertzer and T. Fricke. Chicago: University of Chicago Press.

Kim, J., J. Millen, A. Irwin, and J. Gershman. 2000. *Dying for Growth: Global Inequality and the Health of the Poor*. Monroe, Maine: Common Courage Press.

Klavon, S. L., and G. S. Grubb. 1990. Insertion Site Complications during the First Year of NORPLANT Use. *Contraception* 41(1):27–37.

Kligman, G. 1995. Political Demography: The Banning of Abortion in Ceauseceau's Romania. In *Conceiving the New World Order: The Global Politics of Reproduction*, edited by F. Ginsburg and R. Rapp. Berkeley: University of California Press.

Koalisyon 28 Jiye Chalmay Peral. 1991. NORPLANT: "Piki 5 an." Planing Familyal Pèpè nan Peyi Dayiti. New York: Koalisyon 28 Jiye Chalmay Peral.

Kreager, P. 1982. Demography in Situ. *Population and Development Review* 8(2):237–266.

———. 2004. Objectifying Demographic Identities. In *Categories and Contexts–Anthropological and Historical Studies in Critical Demography*, edited by S. Szreter, H. Sholkamy, and A. Dharmalingam Oxford: Oxford University Press.

Lacombe, R. 1977. La république d'Haïti. *Notes et études documentaires no. 44361*. Paris: La Documentation Française.

Laguerre, M. 1978. The Impact of Migration on the Haitian Family and Household Organization. In *Family and Kinship in Middle America and the Caribbean*, edited by A. Marks and R. Romer.

Leiden, Netherlands: University of the Netherlands Antilles and the Department of Caribbean Studies at the Royal Institute of Linguistics and Anthropology.

———. 1987. Afro-Caribbean Folk Medicine. South Hadley, Mass: Bergin and Garvey.

Lancaster, R., and M. di Leonardo. 1997. *The Gender and Sexuality Reader; Culture, History, Political Economy*. New York: Routledge.

Lappe, F., and R. Schurman. 1990. *Taking Population Seriously*. San Francisco: Institute for Food and Policy Development.

LaRamée, P. 1994. North American Congress on Latin America Observers' Delegation to Haiti. NACLA Haiti Delegation Report. New York: NACLA.

Lazarus, E. 1988. Theoretical Considerations for the Study of the Doctor-Patient Relationship: Implications of a Perinatal Study. *Medical Anthropology Quarterly* 2(1):34–58.

Lerebours, G., and M. A. Canez. 1992. Migration à la Cité Soleil. Unpublished manuscript. Port-au-Prince: Institut Haïtien de l'Enfance.

Lesthaeghe, R. 1980. On the Social Control of Human Reproduction. *Population and Development Review* 6(4):527–548.

Libète. 1995a. Prezidan Aristid Nan Site Soley. *Libète*, 123:1, Port-au-Prince.

———. 1995b. Gen 4 Nouvo Minis nan Gouvenman Michel la. *Libète*, 151:2. Port-au-Prince.

Library of Congress Country Studies. n.d. *Haiti: Decades of instability 1843–1915.* Section 1 of 1. http://lcweb2.loc.gov/cgi-bin/query/r?frd/cstdy:@field(DOCID+ht0022).

Lock, M., and P. A. Kaufert, eds. 1998. *Pragmatic Women and Body Politics.* Cambridge: Cambridge University Press.

Lowenthal, I. 1984. Two to Tango: Haitian Men and Family Planning. Paper submitted to USAID/Haiti Public Health Office.

———. 1987. Marriage is 20, Children are 21: The Cultural Construction of Conjugality and the Family in Rural Haiti. PhD dissertation, Johns Hopkins University.

Maine, D., A. Rosenfield, et al. 1987. Prevention of Maternal Deaths in Developing Countries: Program Options and Practical Considerations. Paper prepared for the International Safe Motherhood Conference, Nairobi.

Maingrette, A. 1995. Historique de la Cité Soleil. *Le Nouvelliste*, 26 July. Port-au-Prince.

Mamdani, M. 1972. *The Myth of Population Control: Family, Caste, and Class in an Indian Village.* New York: Monthly Review Press.

Marcus, G., and M. Fischer. 1986. *Anthropology as Cultural Critique: An Experimental Moment in the Human Sciences.* Chicago: University of Chicago Press.

Markham, R. B., J. Coberly, A. Ruff, D. Hoover, et al. 1994. Maternal IgG1 and IgA Antibody to V3 Loop Consensus Sequence and Maternal-Infant HIV–1 Transmission. *Lancet* 343(8894):390–391.

Marquez, S. 1995. Reuters News Service Press Dispatch. Reuters 23:17, 21 October.

Mason, K. O. 1987. The Impact of Women's Social Position on Fertility in Developing Countries. *Sociological Forum* 2(4):718–745.

———. 1995. Gender and Demographic Change: What Do We Know? In *International Union for the Scientific Study of Population.* Belgium.

Mason, K. O., and A. Malhotra Taj. 1986. Differences between Women's and Men's Reproductive Goals in Developing Countries. *Population and Development Review* 13(4): 611–638.

Maternowska, M. C. 1986. Plannin Mwen Se Grenn Nan: Ou Listwa Reyèl Nan Site Simon. Masters Thesis, University of Michigan.

———. 2005. Haiti Eyes. The Lives Column, *New York Times Magazine*, 24 July 2005, Section 6: 66.

May, J., G. Maynard-Tucker, and J. Guengant. 1991a. Hope for Family Planning in Haiti? Unpublished manuscript draft.

May, J., E. Murphy, and G. Murphy. 1991b. Options II Strategy for Assistance in Haiti. Washington, D.C.: Futures Group. Unpublished manuscript, August.

Maynard-Tucker, G. 1991. The Mystery Client: A Method of Evaluating Quality of Care of the Family Planning Services in the Haitian Private Sector. Paper presented at 1991 NCIH International Health Conference, Crystal City, Md.

McAllister, E. 2002. *Rara!* Berkeley: University of California Press.

McFadyen, D. 1995. FRAPH and CDS: Two Faces of Oppression in Haiti. In *Haiti, Dangerous Crossroads. North American Congress on Latin America (NACLA)*, edited by D. McFadyen, P. LaRamée, M. Fried, and F. Rosen. Boston, Mass.: South End Press.

McNicoll, G. 1978. On Fertility Policy Research (Notes and Commentary). *Population and Development Review* 4(4):681–693.

———. 1983. The Nature of Institutional and Community Effects on Demographic Behavior: An Overview. Working papers no. 101, Center for Policy Studies. New York: Population Council.

———. 1993a. Demography in the Unmaking of Civil Society. Working paper no. 79. New York: Population Council.

———. 1993b. Institutional Analysis of Fertility. Revised text of paper presented at series on Population, Environment, and Development. Beijer Institute, Royal Swedish Academy of Sciences, Stockholm, October.

Medecins Sans Frontieres. 2005. Caught in Haiti's Crossfire. http://www.msf.org/ msfinternational/invoke.cfm?component=article&objectid=475034A7-E018-0C72-0937EF934E4E981B&method=full_html.

MICIVIH (OAS-UN International Civilian Mission in Haiti). 1995. Reflections on the Evolution of Human Rights in Haiti. Interview with Javier Zuniga, Human Rights Director, 26 October. MICIVIH News, English/French, 2 pages.

Mintz, S. 1974. *Caribbean Transformations.* Chicago: Aldine.

Mitchell, T. 2002. *Rule of Experts: Egypt, Techno-Politics and Modernity.* Berkeley: University of California Press.

Molyneux, M. 1985. Mobilization without Emancipation? Women's Interests, the State and Revolution in Nicaragua. *Feminist Studies* 11(2):227–254.

Moral, P. 1961. *Le paysan haitien.* Port-au-Prince: Les Editions Fardin.

Morgan, L. 1987. Dependency Theory in Political Economy of Health: An Anthropological Critique. *Medical Anthropology Quarterly* 1(2):131–154.

Morgan, L. N. 1989. "Political Will" and Community Participation in Costa Rican Primary Health Care. *Medical Anthropology Quarterly* 3(3):232–245.

———. 1993. *Community Participation in Health: The Politics of Primary Care in Costa Rica.* Cambridge: Cambridge University Press.

Morton, A. 1997. Haiti: NGO Sector Study. Washington, D.C., World Bank.

Morsy, S. A. 1993. Bodies of Choice: Norplant Experimental Trials on Egyptian Women. In *Norplant under Her Skin,* edited by B. Mintzes, A. Hardon, and J. Hanhart. Amsterdam: Women's Health Action Foundation (WEMOS).

———. 1995. Deadly Reproduction among Egyptian Women: Maternal Mortality and the Medicalization of Population Control. In *Conceiving the New World Order: The Global Politics of Reproduction,* edited by F. Ginsburg and R. Rapp. Berkeley: University of California Press.

Mott, F. L., and S. Mott. 1985. Household Fertility Decisions in West Africa: A Comparison of Male and Female Survey Results. *Studies in Family Planning* 16(2):88–99.

MSF (Médecins sans Frontières). 2005. The Humanitarian Situation in Haiti: A Statement Delivered by Dr. Christophe Fournier, MSF, to the United Nations Security Council "Arria Formula" Meeting, April 8. http://www.doctorswithoutborders.org/publications/ speeches/2005/christophe_fournier_hhaiti_aria.cfm.

MSH (Management Sciences for Health). 1999. HS 2004 Impact Survey for 1998. Port-au-Prince: MSH HS–2004 Project.

Murray, G. F. 1972. Culture and Fertility Field Work in Haiti Relevant to Family Planning: Progress Report. Unpublished manuscript. Ann Arbor: University of Michigan.

NACLA (North American Congress on Latin America). 1994. Two Faces of Oppression in Haiti. *Report on the Americas.* March/April 27(5):5.

Nag, M., ed. 1975. *Population and Social Organization.* The Hague: Mouton.

———. 1989. Political Awareness as a Factor in Accessibility of Health Services: A Case Study of Rural Kerala and West Bengal. Working papers no. 3. New York: Population Council.

Nag, M., and N. Kak. 1984. Demographic Transition in a Punjab Village. *Population and Development Review* 10(4):661–678.

Nairn, A. 1994. Behind Haiti's Paramilitaries. *The Nation*, 24 October, 18–21.

Nanda, P. 2002. Gender Dimensions of User Fees: Implications for Women's Utilization of Health Care. *Reproductive Health Matters* 10(20):127–134.

Neptune-Anglade, Mireille. 1986. *L'Autre Mitié du Developpement*. Paris: Diffusion Karthala.

———. 1995. *Fanm Aisyen an Chif.* Port-au-Prince: Comité Inter-Agences Femmes et Développement (CIFD) en Haiti.

New York Times. 2003. The War against Women. Editorials/Letters, *New York Times*, 12 January.

Nicholls, D. 1979. *From Dessalines to Duvalier: Race, Colour, and National Independence in Haiti*. Cambridge: Cambridge University Press.

Nichter, M., and E. Cartwright. 1991. Saving the Children for the Tobacco Industry. *Medical Anthropology Quarterly* 5(3):236–256.

Nifong, C. 1994. US Groups Rally to Support Haitian Women. *Christian Science Monitor*, 30 November, 12.

NLC (National Labor Committee). 1993. Haiti after the Coup: Sweatshop or Real Development? Special Delegation Report of the National Labor Committee Education Fund in Support of Worker and Human Rights in Central America. New York.

Norton, M. 2003. Bus, Taxi Drivers Call Strike in Haiti. *Associated Press*, 7 January.

Notestein, F. 1953. Economic Problems of Population Change. In *Proceedings of the International Conference of Agricultural Economists*. London: Oxford University Press.

Nouvelliste, Le. 1996. Le CDS pourrait fermer ses portes à Cité Soleil. Les Ramous de l'Actualité. *Nouvelliste* 35(147):1.

Okediji, F. O. 1975. Socioeconomic Status and Attitudes to Public Health Problems in the Western State: A Case Study of Ibadan. In *J. Population Growth and Socio-economic Change in West Africa*, edited by Caldwell. New York: Columbia University Press/ Population Council.

Olibrice, Z. 1979. *Approche sociologique de l'action communautaire de l'eglise catholique dans la communauté de Brooklyn* (Haiti). Port-au-Prince: Faculté des Sciences Humaines.

Oppong, C. 1983. Women's Roles, Opportunity Costs, and Fertility. In *Determinants of Fertility in Developing Countries*, edited by R. Bulato and R. Lee. New York: Academic Press.

PAHO (Pan American Health Organization). 2004. The Haiti Crisis: Health Risks. http://www.paho.org/English/DD/PED/HaitiHealthImpact.htm.

PAI (Population Action International). 2001. How Slower Population Growth Contributed to the Asian Miracle. PAI Fact Sheet. Washington, D.C.

Paley, J. 2001. *Marketing Democracy: Power and Social Movements in Post-Dictatorship Chile*. Berkeley: University of California Press.

Panikar, P. G. 1979. Resources Not the Constraint on Health Improvement: A Case Study in Kerala. *Economic and Political Weekly* 14(44):1803–1809.

Parker, R., R. M. Barbosa, and P. Aggleton. 2000. *Framing the Sexual Subject: The Politics of Gender, Sexuality, and Power*. Berkeley: University of California Press.

Petchesky, R. 1998. Introduction. In *Negotiating Reproductive Rights: Women's Perspectives across Countries and Cultures*. London: Zed Books.

———. 2000. Sexual Rights: Inventing a Concept, Mapping and International Practice. In *Framing the Sexual Subject. The Politics of Gender, Sexuality, and Power*, edited by R. Parker, R. M. Barbosa, and P. Aggleton. Berkeley: University of California Press.

Pfeiffer, J. 2002. African Independent Churches in Mozambique: Healing the Afflictions of Inequality. *Medical Anthropology Quarterly*, 16(2):176–199.

———. 2004a. Condom Social Marketing, Pentecostalism, and Structural Adjustment in Mozambique: A Clash of AIDS Prevention Messages. *Medical Anthropology Quarterly* 18(1):77–103 .

———. 2004b. International NGOs in the Mozambique Health Sector. In *Unhealthy Health Policy: A Critical Anthropological Examination*, Edited by A. Castro and M. Singer. Walnut Creek, Cal.: Altamira Press.

Philippe, J. and J. B. Romain. 1979. Indisposition in Haiti. *Social Science and Medicine* 13B:129–133.

Pierre-Pierre, G. 1995. Haiti Task Force, Battling for Women's Rights. *New York Times*, 9 September, 2.

PIH (Partners in Health). 2004. *Haiti: STD Program.* PIH/STD Screening and Treatment Program. http://www.pih.org/wherewework/haiti/std.html.

Pincus, G., C. Garcia, J. Rock, M. Paniagua, A. Pendleton, F. Laraque, et al. 1959. Effectiveness of an Oral Contraceptive. *Science* 134(10 July):81–83.

Polgar, S. 1971. Culture, History and Population Dynamics. In *Culture and Population: A Collection of Current Studies*, edited by S. Polgar. Chapel Hill: Carolina Population Center, University of North Carolina.

———. 1972. Population History and Population Policies from an Anthropological Perspective. *Current Anthropology* 12:203–211.

Polgreen, L. 2004. Deepening Poverty Breeds Desperation in Haiti. *New York Times, International Section/Americas.* http://nytimes.com/2004/05/05/international/americas/ 05hait.html.

POLICY Project. n.d. Haiti. http://www.policyproject.com/countries.cfm?country=Haiti.

Population Council. 2002. Using Men as Community-Based Distributors of Condoms. *Frontiers in Reproductive Health.* Program brief no. 2. Washington, D.C.: Population Council.

Potter, J. E., M. Ordonez, and R. A. Measham. 1976. The Rapid Decline in Colombian Fertility. *Population and Development Review* 2(3/4), September–December:509–528.

PPFA (Planned Parenthood Federation of America). n.d. The Global Gag Rule. http://www. plannedparenthood.org/gag/.

Prengaman, P. 2004. Haiti's New Prime Minister Is Sworn In. Associated Press via *Washington Times*, 13 March. http://www.freerepublic.com/focus/news/1096921/posts.

Presser, H. B. 1997. Demography, Feminism and the Science-Policy Nexus. *Population and Development Review* 23(2):295–331.

Pulerwitz, J., S. Gortmaker, and W. DeJong. 2000. Measuring Sexual Relationship Power in HIV/STD Research. *Sex Roles* 42(7/8):637.

Qadeer I. and N. Visvanathan. 2004. How Healthy Are Health and Population Policies? In *The Indian Experience in Unhealthy Health Policy: A Critical Anthropological Examination*, edited by A. Castro and M. Singer. Walnut Creek, Cal.: Altamira Press.

Racine, M. B. 1994. The Long Journey toward Freedom. *Roots* 1(3):7–12.

Renne, E. P. 1995. Houses, Fertility and the Nigerian Land Use Act. *Population and Development Review* 21(1):113–126.

———. 2003. *Population and Progress in a Yoruba Town.* Vancouver: University of British Columbia Press.

Reuters. 1995. Car in Tipper Gore's Motorcade Stoned in Haiti. *Washington Post*, 16 October.

Richey, L. 1999a. "Development," Gender and Family Planning: Population Policies and the Tanzanian National Population Policy. PhD dissertation, Department of Political Science, University of North Carolina at Chapel Hill.

———. 1999b. Family Planning and the Politics of Population in Tanzania: International to Local Discourse. *Journal of African Studies* 37(3):457–487.

———. 2002. Is Overpopulation Still the Problem? Global Discourse and Reproductive Health Challenges in the Time of HIV/AIDS. *Center for Development.* Working paper 02.1. Copenhagen, January.

Ridgeway, J. 1994. C'est plus ça change. *Village Voice*, 1 March, 14–15.

Rosenthal, S. M. 1999. Depo-Provera WebMD Medical Reference from *The Gynecological Sourcebook*. http://my.webmd.com/content/article/4/1680_50968.htm.

Ross, J., and E. Frankenberg. 1993. *Findings from Two Decades of Family Planning Research*. New York: Population Council.

Ross, J., J. S. Willard, and A. Willard. 2000. *Profiles for Family Planning and Reproductive Health Programs 116 Countries*. Glastonbury, Conn.: Futures Group International.

Rouzier, M. N. 1998. *Plantes médicinales d'Haïti*. Quebec: Editions Regain/Les Editions de CIDIHCA.

Rubin, G. 1975. The Traffic in Women: Notes on the Political Economy of Sex. In *Toward an Anthropology of Women*, edited by R. Reiter. New York: Monthly Review.

Save the Children. 2003. *The Mothers' Index and Country Ratings*. 4th ed. http://www.savethechildren.org/sowm2003/MothersIndex.pdf.

Scheper-Hughes, N. 1992. *Death without Weeping: The Violence of Everyday Life in Brazil*. Berkeley: University of California Press.

———. 1997. Demography without Numbers. In *Anthropological Demography*, edited by D. I. Kertzer and T. Fricke. Chicago: University of Chicago Press.

———. 2002. The Ends of the Body: Commodity Fetishism and the Global Traffic in Organs, *SAIS Review* 22(1, Winter–Spring):61–80.

Scheper-Hughes, N., and M. Lock. 1986. Speaking "Truth" to Illness: Metaphors, Reification and a Pedagogy for Patients. *Medical Anthropology Quarterly* 17(5):137–140.

———. 1987. The Mindful Body: A Prolegomenon to Future Work in Medical Anthropology. *Medical Anthropology Quarterly* 1:1.

Schoepf, B. 1988. Women, AIDS, and Economic Crisis in Central Africa. *Canadian Journal of African Studies* 22(3):625–644.

Schuller, M. 2003. A Volatile 200-Year Ménage-à-Trois: Global Forces, the State, and Local Civic Activity in Haiti. Unpublished paper, submitted to review, Ferdinand Braudel Center, University of California, Santa Barbara.

Schwartz, T. T. 2000. Children Are the Wealth of the Poor: High Fertility and the Organization of Labor in the Rural Economy of Jean Rabel, Haiti., PhD dissertation, University of Florida.

Scott, D. 2005. The Lucrative Business of Death. An Analysis of Planned Parenthood Federation of America Inc.'s Annual Report (2003–2004). http://www.fightpp.org/downloads/pubs/Winter%20-%20ws.pdf. Special Reports. Winter Life Decisions International (viii).

Sealy, G. 2005. An Epidemic Failure: Whatever Happened to Bush's Pledge to Combat AIDS in Africa? Rolling Stone. http://www.rollingstone.com/politics/story/_/id/7371950?pageid=rs.Politics&pageregion=single1&rnd=1123383648312&has-player=false.

Sen, A. 1994. Population: Delusion and Reality. *New York Review of Books* 41(15):62–71.

———. 1999. *Development as Freedom*. New York: Alfred Knopf.

Sen, G., A. Germain, and L. Chen, eds. 1994. *Population Policies Reconsidered: Health, Empowerment and Rights*. Boston: Harvard School of Public Health.

Sen, G., and R. C. Snow. 1994. *Power and Decision: The Social Control of Reproduction*. Harvard Series on Population and International Health. Cambridge: Harvard University Press.

SEP (Secrétairerie d'Etat à la Population). 2000. *Politique nationale de population*. Port-au-Prince: Ministère de la Santé Publique et de la Population.

Setel, P. 1999. *A Plague of Paradoxes: AIDS, Culture, and Demography in Northern Tanzania*. Chicago: University of Chicago Press.

Shakow, A. 2003. An Inter-American Emergency. *PIH Bulletin*. Boston: Partners in Health, Winter, 2.

Simmons, R., and C. Elias. 1994. The Study of Client-Provider Interactions: A Review of Methodological Issues. *Studies in Family Planning* 25(1):1–17.

Singer, M. 1986. Developing a Critical Perspective in Medical Anthropology. *Medical Anthropology Quarterly* 17(5, November):128–129.

——. 1995. Beyond the Ivory Tower: Critical Praxis in Medical Anthropology. *Medical Anthropology Quarterly* 9(1):80–106.

——. 2003. Can There Be a Critical Medical Applied Anthropology? *Newsletter of the Society for Applied Anthropology*. http://www.sfaa.net/Newsletter-2003/css/Newsletter_2003_5.htm.

Singer, M., and H. Baer, 1995. *Critical Medical Anthropology*. Amityville, N.Y.: Baywood.

Singer, M., and A. Castro. 2004. Introduction: Anthropology and Health Policy: A Critical Perspective. In *Unhealthy Health Policy: A Critical Anthropological Examination*, edited by A. Castro and M. Singer. Walnut Creek, Cal.: Altamira Press.

Smith, J. M. 2001. *When the Hands Are Many: Community Organization and Social Change in Rural Haiti*. Ithaca: Cornell University Press.

Smith, J. 1990. Strategy for the Population Sector. USAID/Haiti. 1990–1992. Washington, DC:USAID.

Smith Fawzi, M. C., W. Lambert, J. M. Singer, Y. Tanagho, F. Léandre, P. Nevil, D. Bertrand, M. S. Claude, J. Bertrand, M. Louissant, L. Joanis, J. S. Mukherjee, S. Goldie, J. J. Salazar, and P. E. Farmer, 2005. Factors Associated with Forced Sex among Women in Rural Haiti: Implications for the Prevention of HIV and other STDs. *Social Science and Medicine* 60(4):679–689.

Sneider, D. 2005. Kidnappings Plague Haiti. *Mercury News*, 20 June. http://www.mercurynews.com/mld/mercurynews/news/columnists/daniel_sneider/11938634.htm.

Sobo, A. 1993. *One Blood: The Jamaican Body*. Albany: State University of New York Press.

Stebbins, K. R. 2001. Going Like GangBusters: Transnational Tobacco Companies "Making a Killing" in South America. *Medical Anthropology Quarterly* 15(2):147–170.

Stoler, A. L. 1991. Carnal Knowledge and Imperial Power: Gender, Race and Morality in Colonial Asia. In *Gender at the Crossroads of Knowledge: Feminist Anthropology in the Post-Modern Era*, edited by Micaela Di Leonardo. Berkeley: University of California Press.

Stopka, T., M. Singer, C. Santelices, and J. Eiserman. 2003. Public Health Interventionists, Penny Capitalists, or Sources of Risk? Assessing Street Syringe Sellers in Hartford, Connecticut. *Substance Use and Misuse* 38(9):1339–1370.

Szreter, S. 1993. The Idea of Demographic Transition and the Study of Fertility Change. *Population and Development Review* 19(4):659–693.

Szreter, S., H. Sholkamy, and A. Dharmalingam. 2004. Editors' Introduction (Chapter 12). In *Categories and Contexts—Anthropological and Historical Studies in Critical Demography*. Oxford: Oxford University Press.

Tafforeau, J. 1989. Operations Research Project for Improvement of Accessibility to Family Planning Services in Cité Soleil. Unpublished report. Port-au-Prince: Columbia University.

Tafforeau, J., J. Allman, and S. Allman. 1985. Attitudes and Acceptance of DMPA in Rural Haiti. Paper presented to the American Public Health Association Meeting. Washington, D.C., November.

Tafforeau, J., and R. Boulos. 1986. Acceptabilité du DEPOPROVERA en Haïti. Paper prepared for the *National Council for International Health*. Washington, D.C., June.

TAG (Technique d'Administration, d'Animation et de Gestion). 2001. L'Avortement en Haïti et ses conséquences: Analyse de la situation. Unpublished report. Port-au-Prince.

Time. 1994. Cité Soleil Inferno. *Time Magazine* (International 10th edition), 11 January.

Todd, A. 1989. *Intimate Adversaries: Cultural Conflict between Doctors and Women Patients*. Philadelphia: University of Pennsylvania Press.

Towghi, F. 2004. Shifting Policies toward Traditional Midwives: The Implications for Reproductive Health Care in Pakistan. In *Unhealthy Health Policy: A Critical Anthropological Examination*, edited by A. Castro and M. Singer. Walnut Creek, Cal.: Altamira press.

Trouillot, M. 1990. *Haiti: State against Nation. The Origins and Legacy of Duvalierism.* New York: Monthly Review Press.

———. 1995a. *Silencing the Past: Power and the Production of History.* Boston: Beacon Press.

———. 1995b. Haiti's Nightmare and the Lessons of History. In *Haiti, Dangerous Crossroads*, edited by E. McFadyen, P. LaRamée, M. Fried, and F. Rosen. North American Congress on Latin America (NACLA). Boston: South End Press.

———. 2001. The Anthropology of the State in the Age of Globalization. *Current Anthropology* 42(1):125–138.

UCSF (University of California San Francisco). 2003. Family PACT Program Report. FY 2001/2002. A Report to the State of California Department of Health Services, Office of Family Planning. Unpublished report 30 June.

UNDP (United Nations Development Program). 1994. Human Development Report. Oxford: Oxford University Press.

———. 2003. Human Development Report 2000. New York: Oxford University Press.

UNFPA (United Nations Fund for Population Activities). 1994. New Study Finds 50 Percent Abortion Rate among Haitian Teenagers. Briefing paper no. 1. Port-au-Prince: Fonds des Nations Unies pour la Population.

———. 2001. Maternal Mortality in 2001: Estimates Developed by WHO, UNICEF and UNFPA. http://www.childinfo.org/eddb/mat_mortal/.

UNICEF (United Nations Children's Fund). 1994a. Analyse de la situation des femmes et des enfants en Haiti (periode 1980–1993). Port-au-Prince: UNICEF.

———. 1994b. The State of the World's Children. Oxford: Oxford University Press.

———. 2003a. At a Glance: Haiti—The Big Picture. http://unicef.org/infobycountry/ haiti.html.

———. 2003b. Statistics: Maternal Mortality. News as of October 2003: The Challenge. http:// www.childinfo.org/eddb/mat_mortal/.

———. 2004. Monitoring and Statistics, At a Glance: Haiti. http://www.unicef.org/ infobycountry/haiti_statistics.html.

United Nations. 1991. The World's Women 1970–1990: Trends and Statistics. *Social Statistics and Indicators*. Series K (8). New York: United Nations.

USAID (United States Agency for International Development). 1991. Overview of A.I.D. Population Assistance. Office of Population, Agency for International Development. April.

———. 1993. Executive Summary, PFPS project no. 521–0189, Second Interim Evaluation, Haiti. Port-au-Prince: USAID Health and Family Planning Division.

———. 1999. FY 2001 Results Review and Resources Request (R4). Arlington, Va., March.

———. 2000. Population and Health. http://www.usaid.gov/ht/health.html.

———. 2002. Haiti: Activity Data Sheet. http://www.usaid.gov/pubs/cbj2002/lac/ht/521-003. html.

Waitzkin, H. 1991. *The Politics of Medical Encounters: How Doctors Deal with Social Problems.* New Haven: Yale University Press.

Walton, D., P. Farmer, W. Lambert, F. Léandre, S. Koenig and J. Mukherjee. 2004. Integrated HIV Prevention and Care Strengthens Primary Health Care: Lessons from Rural Haiti. *Journal of Public Health Policy* 25(2):137–158.

Wang, G., and V. Pillai. 2001. Women's Reproductive Health: A Gender Sensitive Human Rights Approach. *Acta Sociológica* 44:231.

Ward, E. G., W. B. Disch, J. A. Levy, and J. J. Schensul. 2004. Perception of HIV/AIDS Risk among Urban, Low-Income Senior Housing Residents. *AIDS Education and Prevention*, 16(6):571–588.

Ward, M. 1986. *Poor Women, Powerful Men*. Boulder, Col.: Westview Press.

Warwick, Donald, P. 1982. *Bitter Pills: Population Policies and Their Implementation in Eight Developing Countries*. Cambridge: Cambridge University Press.

Watkins, S. C. 1993. If All We Knew about Women Was What We Read in Demography, What Would We Know? *Demography* 30(4):551–577.

Weinreb, A. A. 2001. First Politics, Then Culture. Accounting for Ethnic Differences in Demographic Behavior in Kenya. *Population and Development Review* 27(3):437–467.

WHO (World Health Organization). 2001. Maternal Mortality in 1995. United Nations Children's Fund and the United Nations Population Fund, http://ddp-ext.worldbank.org/ext/GMIS/gdmis.do?siteID=Z&contentID=Content_#68menuId=LNAVoIHOMEI.

Wilentz, A. 1989. *The Rainy Season*. New York: Simon and Schuster.

Wolf, E. 1969. American Anthropologists and American Society. In *Reinventing Anthropology*, edited by D. Hymes. New York: Vintage Press.

———. 1982. *Europe and the People without History*. Berkeley: University of California Press.

World Bank. 1993a. Effective Family Planning Programs. Washington, D.C.: World Bank.

———. 1993b. World Development Report. New York: Oxford University Press.

———. 1998. Sri Lanka's Health Sector: Achievements and Challenges. World Bank Group. http://lnweb18.worldbank.org/sar/sa.nsf/0/c5395c25703aabdd8525687e005bd666?OpenDocument.

Wyon, J. B., and J. E. Gordon. 1971. *The Khanna Study*. Cambridge: Harvard University Press.

Zapata, C., A. Rebolledo, E. Atalah, B. Newman, and M. King. 1992. The Influence of Social and Political Violence on the Risk of Pregnancy Complications. *American Journal of Public Health* 82(5):685–690.

Zierler, S., and N. Krieger. 1998. HIV Infection in Women: Social Inequalities as Determinants of Risk. *Critical Public Health* 8(1):13–32.

INDEX

ABOUT THE AUTHOR

M. CATHERINE MATERNOWSKA holds dual faculty appointments as assistant professor within the departments of obstetrics and gynecology and reproductive sciences as well as anthropology, history, and social medicine at the University of California, San Francisco. Her research examines the impact of sexually transmitted infections, poor prenatal care, and the absence of good obstetric and gynecological services on the health of women and adolescents living in poverty. She has conducted research in California and Mexico among migrant workers, analyzing issues of gender, power, and access to health care. Her current research focuses on maternal mortality and access to health care and the political economy of health among adolescent HIV/AIDS orphans living in Zimbabwe and Tanzania. Dr. Maternowska studied social geography and economics at the London School of Economics and Political Science (BSc 1983), population and international health at the University of Michigan (MPH 1986), and medical anthropology at Columbia University (PhD 1996).